Chronic Disorders
and the Family

ABOUT THE EDITORS

Froma Walsh, PhD, is Associate Professor of both Social Work and Psychiatry at the University of Chicago. She is affiliated with the Family Institute of Chicago, Northwestern University Medical Center. Dr. Walsh is especially known for her internationally acclaimed collection, *Normal Family Processes*. Her latest book, *Treating Severely Dysfunctional Families*, will be released soon.

Carol M. Anderson, PhD, is Professor of Psychiatry at the University of Pittsburgh and Director of the Family Institute of Pittsburgh. She is the President-elect of the American Family Therapy Association, author of numerous influential publications, including her most recent book, *Schizophrenia and the Family*, co-authored with Reiss and Hogarty.

Chronic Disorders and the Family

Froma Walsh
Carol Anderson
Editors

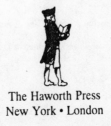

The Haworth Press
New York • London

Chronic Disorders and the Family has also been published as *Journal of Psychotherapy & the Family*, Volume 3, Number 3 Fall 1987.

The Haworth Press, Inc., 12 West 32 Street, New York, NY 10001
EUROSPAN/Haworth, 3 Henrietta Street, London WC2E 8LU England

Library of Congress Cataloging-in-Publication Data

Chronic disorders and the family.

Has also been published as Journal of psychotherapy & the family ; v. 3, no. 3 (Fall 1987).
Includes bibliographies.
1. Family psychotherapy. 2 Mental illness—Treatment. I. Walsh, Froma.
II. Anderson, Carol M., 1939- . [DNLM: 1. Family Therapy. 2. Mental Disorders—therapy.
W1 JO859C v. 3 no. 3 / WM 430.5.F2 C557]
RC488.5.C47 1987 616.89'156 87-31196
ISBN 0-86656-700-3
ISBN 0-86656-926-X (pbk.)

Chronic Disorders
and the Family

CONTENTS

FOREWORD

This special issue focuses on the treatment of severe and chronic mental and physical illnesses from a family systems perspective.

The co-editors of this important book, Froma Walsh and Carol Anderson are both internationally known and respected scholars and psychotherapists. Both have recently written important books on the focus of their collaborative effort. Dr. Walsh is an associate professor of both social work and psychiatry at the University of Chicago and is also affiliated with the Family Institute of Chicago, Northwestern University Medical Center. She is especially known for her internationally acclaimed collection, *Normal Family Processes*. Her latest book, *Treating Severely Dysfunctional Families*, will be released soon.

Dr. Anderson is a professor of psychiatry at the University of Pittsburgh and Director of the Family Institute of Pittsburgh. She is the President-elect of the American Family Therapy Association, author of numerous influential articles and books, including her recent book, *Schizophrenia and the Family*, co-authored with Reiss and Hogarty.

In the first article the editors state that they have assembled this special volume to encourage psychotherapists to compare and contrast the various treatment perspectives and approaches available in this area. Moreover they have attempted to provide a forum for leading scholars to promote and explicate their orientation to one or more disorders vis-à-vis the family.

Because of their knowledge and leadership of this important area, they have attracted to this collection an impressive group of papers written by highly respected scholar-clinicians: Craig Everett, Sandra Volgy, Michael Rohrbaugh, Glenn Shean, Richard Schwartz,

1

John Schwartzman, Peter Steinglass, Mary Horan, John Rolland, and Evan Imber-Black.

Here these scholar-practitioners address fundamental issues in psychotherapy practice. The collective effort, among other things, is to help their colleagues to more effectively measure and treat one of the oldest and most difficult set of presenting problems: severe, chronic disorders. Disorders discussed directly include schizophrenia, clinical depression, borderline disorders, anxiety disorders, particularly agoraphobia, eating disorders, substance abuse, and chronic medical illnesses. In addition to addressing these specific disorders, several papers effectively summarize and synthesize the various issues surrounding this emerging sub-speciality of family treatment of chronic mental disorders.

Charles R. Figley, PhD

Chronic Disorders and Families:
An Overview

Froma Walsh
Carol Anderson

The papers in this volume present recent developments in clinical research and theory on the role of the family in understanding and treating severe and chronic mental and physical illnesses. The goal is to increase awareness of the problems facing families coping with all severe disorders, as well as issues specific to particular disorders. Each of the first six papers presents a review of the most recent knowledge and practice developments within representative major psychiatric diagnostic groups, including schizophrenia (Walsh), depression (Anderson), borderline disorders (Everett & Volgy), anxiety disorders (Rohrbaugh & Shean), eating disorders (Schwartz), and substance abuse (Schwartzman). The next two papers (Steinglass & Horan; Rolland) address the role of the family in chronic medical conditions, moving toward an integrative view of the family and chronic illness. The final paper (Imber-Black) examines the difficulties families confront in transactions with health care systems in the treatment of chronic disorders.

This collection was assembled to encourage clinicians to compare and contrast the various perspectives and approaches to intervention that have characterized recent developments in understanding and treating specific disorders. As important as it is to construct meaningful categories that distinguish a particular disorder from others, it is equally important to gain a broader perspective about family issues in a range of severe and chronic disorders. To do so, it is also important to become more aware of the common experiences of patients and their families struggling with chronic psychiatric and medical disor-

Froma Walsh, PhD, is Associate Professor at the University of Chicago and is on the faculty of the Family Institute of Chicago. Carol Anderson, PhD, is Professor, Department of Psychiatry, University of Pittsburgh, and Director of the Family Institute of Pittsburgh.

3

ders. This process will promote a better understanding of the contribution of the family and broader social context to the course of major disorders as well as the reciprocal impact of severe dysfunction and chronicity on family functioning. This introductory paper offers an overview of emerging, and as yet divergent, perspectives on severe disorders and the family. It will trace developments in the family field which have led to the adoption of a systems paradigm and suggest directions for future research, theory building and practice.

THE DEVELOPMENT OF A SYSTEMIC ORIENTATION

Traditionally, health professionals have approached chronic mental and physical disorders from an individual perspective. Attempts to understand their development, course, and outcome have tended to focus either on the genetic makeup or on the early developmental history of individual patients and the personality structures or personal attributes that "result." Whether biological or psychodynamic factors were emphasized, the view was likely to be a pessimistic one since in either case, individual destiny was largely predetermined since there were no effective ways of influencing it.

Recent advances in our understanding of biological factors and concommitant innovations in medical and psychiatric treatments have demonstrated that the course of many disorders can be influenced. Simultaneous advances in the conceptualization of social and family variables as important factors in the onset and/or the course of various illnesses have begun to lay the foundation for the development of a genuine systems approach to chronic disorders.

In the research arena, the study of family variables has shifted from a focus on factors which might contribute to the etiology or "origin" of disorders, to attempts to understand the ongoing transactional processes within which individuals and their dysfunctions are currently embedded. The inevitable stresses of family life in general, combined with the particular patterns of past and current adaptation are now examined in attempts to understand how environments may exacerbate or mitigate preexisting biological or genetic vulnerabilities or current stresses. In this process, an increased respect is developing for the reciprocal of processes of influence between patients and their families. In addition to the long recognized impact of families on individuals, there is an increased recognition of the impact of dysfunctional patients on their families — including the impact of the cumulative stress and burden of coping with chronic problems.

These ideas, though not yet fully integrated into our current practices, offer the beginnings of a new paradigm, a bio-psycho-social view for understanding patients in context, and the important role families can play in treating patients with chronic medical and psychiatric disorders.

FROM MIND-BODY SPLIT TO WHOLISTIC PERSPECTIVE

Surveying and comparing family variables in a range of severe and chronic disorders requires a shift away from the traditional mind/body split toward a wholistic perspective. The development of an integrated view of psychiatric and medical disorders requires attention to the reciprocal impact of biological and psychosocial influences. However, despite increased awareness of the complicated, interacting forces between biological and social, family and individual, these ideas are not well integrated into the treatment of patients and their families. In professional circles, there remains a division between those who concentrate on individual biologic or dynamic variables, and those who focus primarily on family variables (Lansky, 1981). All too often, neither group sufficiently recognizes the importance of the contribution of the other set of factors, preventing the development of a truly comprehensive approach which could be adopted by mainstream clinicians to provide more effective interventions.

There is, however, an increasing commitment to the notion of developing programs for families of patients with severe disorders. The movement for deinstitutionalization placed many chronically ill psychiatric patients with their families in the community rather than in hospitals. In psychiatry, this phenomenon was strengthened by policies of utilization review, treatment contracts, and informed consent, all of which emphasize the briefest possible hospital stays. In medicine, health care advances increasingly have resulted in the indefinite extension of the lives of patients who will never be well. In either case, the expectation that families will be the primary caretakers of patients who once required twenty-four hour care by a *group* of professionals has precipitated increased pressure for changes in the support programs and resources provided by hospitals and community health programs.

Perhaps because of these changes, several simultaneous shifts in the attitudes of both clinicians and researchers about families have occurred. There seems to be: (1) greater acceptance of the evidence for the influence of biological variables; (2) increased awareness of the impact of chronic problems and stresses on family functioning; (3) a growing concern about genuinely informed consent and other ethical issues in treatment; and (4) increased awareness of the need to cooperate with consumer groups demanding more respect and information. In summary, the relationship between families and professionals is increasingly one of collaboration and respect. All of these developments have highlighted the problems in psychiatry of diagnosis and its relationship to family variables.

PSYCHIATRY, PATIENT DIAGNOSIS AND THE DSM-III

The tendency toward specialization in the field of mental health has resulted in skewed and fragmented views of the role of the family in chronic disorders. The influence of the medical model and development of the DSM-III have contributed to the tendency to type families according to the particular diagnosis of an identified patient. Funding for clinical research, training, and services is mainly targeted for investigation and treatment of specific disorders, with family research and treatment programs tending to focus exclusively on attempts to isolate particular disorder-specific family patterns. Over time, as funding priorities change and attention shifts to different disorders, there has been a failure to build a cumulative body of knowledge about families across diagnostic categories.

There is considerable controversy concerning issues of family assessment and patient diagnosis, particularly in regard to major psychiatric disorders. Recently, the American Psychiatric Association Task Force for the revision of the DSM-III considered the creation of a family axis for the classification system (Wynne, personal communication). The effort was fraught with difficulties. First, there was reluctance to add any new axes since the present five axes already have proven to be cumbersome for clinicians. Second, the DSM-III was designed primarily as a classification of disorders *within* persons. A family classification system, while clinically useful, was thought by some to be beyond the scope of this categorization of diseases. Others, including some family therapists, objected to the use of codes in Axis I, regarding conditions for attention to treatment that are not individual diagnoses, because such categories are currently not reimbursable. The Task Force therefore moved to redesign Axis IV: (Severity of Psychosocial Stressors) to identify stressors in family systems, work settings, and other social situations. It was decided that a distinction between acute and chronic stressors would be useful, given the literature suggesting that chronic stressors have a long-term psychophysiological influence in setting the stage for illness, whereas acute stressors, such as a family crisis, may have a more immediate impact in triggering symptoms, such as a panic attack. In the DSM-IIIR, the presence of acute events (under six months) and "enduring circumstances" (over six months) are rated from one to seven, with family factors and other content areas to be noted.

An advantage of the plan for the DSM-IIIR is that it will alert clinicians to indications for a family evaluation. A disadvantage is that it does not provide sufficient information to guide plans for family intervention. In response to concern that the term "stressors" implies a causal role in disorders when no such link may exist, the text states explicitly that family or other social processes may be, at least in part, a consequence of the individual member's disorder. Nevertheless, the possible protective contributions that families might make to the patients' illness and its course are not taken into account. Our chief concern is that indications for family evaluation and family intervention would be equated with family pathology and/or perpetuate the presumption of a family causal role in the etiology or maintenance of an individual disorder. In the past, families have been blamed and scapegoated. They have been given the implicit or explicit message that family intervention is recommended *because* they are the cause of a patient's disturbance. It would be far more productive to base the rationale for family intervention on respect for the needs of family members, and the value of the family's collaborative role in improving patient functioning. Any family distress, regardless of origin or type, should be a sufficient indication for evaluation for possible family intervention if we are to be responsive to family as well as patient needs.

The dilemma of the DSM-III may seem irrelevant to many with a family systems orientation. Some such clinicians have rejected the use of diagnostic categories altogether, out of concern that the symptomatic family member should not be scapegoated or encouraged to assume a patient role that reinforces dysfunction and hopelessness about change, or that disregards the complimentary or reinforcing roles of other family members. Some family therapists also regard individual diagnosis as irrelevant to the process of change. A few have gone so far as to propose a single family intervention approach, such as the "invariant prescription" of Selvini Palazzoli (1986), for all families with a severely dysfunctional member, regardless of individual diagnosis or family characteristics.

It is of course important not to reify diagnostic categories in a way that partializes and distorts experience, ignores the diversity and complexity of human experience, scapegoats patients *or* families, or prevents us from seeing common elements inherent in coping with any severe and chronic disorder. Nevertheless, we would argue for the potential value of diagnostic categories where they provide clarifying information and guide effective intervention. In the development of knowledge about severe disorders and their treatment, it is valuable to identify interactional patterns and regularities typically associated with various symptom clusters and with good versus poor outcome. The use of these categories also makes possible the comparison of the results of our interventions with those of other orientations. Without the ability to demonstrate the effectiveness of our work, we are unlikely to survive in an increasingly competitive and skeptical climate.

ASSESSMENT OF FAMILY FUNCTIONING AND FAMILY TYPOLOGIES

The DSM-III experience suggests that it may be more fruitful for family therapists to construct a separate classification system for the assessment of family functioning. However, attempts to construct family typologies based on the psychiatric diagnosis of an individual patient are problematic. First, severity of individual psychopathology cannot be equated with severity of dysfunction in families. In other words, not all families with a chronically disturbed member are severely dysfunctional as a family unit. In fact, given the evidence for a biological component in schizophrenia, affective disorders, substance abuse, and most probably other severe and chronic mental disturbances, family pathology may be neither a necessary nor a sufficient factor for the development of major psychiatric disorders. Certainly, while a role is beginning to be identified in some illnesses, family factors are not seen as vital to the development of most medical disorders. More likely, as has been hypothesized in the stress-vulnerability model (Zubin & Spring, 1977) biological factors probably interact with both the level and mode of family functioning and other stresses impinging on the patient and family. In patients with a stronger genetic loading, or biochemical vulnerability, less severe stress may be necessary to elicit symptoms of the disorder, while patients with less biological vulnerability may require more extreme or prolonged stress for symptoms to appear (Tecce & Cole, 1976).

Family research over the past three decades has found significant associations between a number of family variables and particular patient disorders and outcomes. Findings reviewed in the following papers suggest that certain family interaction patterns are found more frequently for patients with a particular diagnosis than for others. Yet it must be kept in mind that there is no one-to-one correspondence between a specific psychiatric diagnosis and a single family attribute or style (Walsh, 1987). There is considerable diversity among the families of similarly diagnosed individuals in the way they interact, cope, and respond to the patient. Not all individuals with the same symptoms have the same type of family system (Russell, Olson, Sprenkle, & Atilano, 1983). It is important, therefore, not to assume that the family of an individual with a particular disorder has a corresponding pattern of dysfunction. For this reason, we advise against the practice of labeling a family by the diagnosis of an individual member. Just as the term "schizophrenogenic mother" became a pejorative label applied to any mother with a schizophrenic offspring, such terms as "schizophrenic family" or "alcoholic family" stereotype, pathologize and alienate families. Treatment planning should be based on an assessment of the needs of each family member in each family system as well as on the symptoms of the presenting patient (Olson & Walsh, in press).

Another limitation of family typologies based on individual diagnosis is that many families with a severely disturbed member are multiproblem families, characterized by a number of dysfunctional patterns and more than one "diagnosable" member. Since most research and clinical attention focuses on the "identified" patient, the disturbances of other members that are undiagnosed or that are only evident at another point in time are ignored. This poses a dilemma for categorizing families. For example, in a schizophrenia research program (Walsh, in press), one family was assigned to the "disturbed nonschizophrenic" control group because their hospitalized son was diagnosed as manic-depressive. Two years later, the subject's brother was hospitalized with a diagnosis of chronic schizophrenia. When this occurred, did the family change from an "affective disorder family" to a "schizophrenic family?" Should they be recategorized as a "family of a schizophrenic?" Should they be measured twice in two separate categories for each son? Should they be ruled out of the study altogether because they are not a "pure" type? Would any of these "solutions" contribute to our understanding of family variables?

The construction of family typologies is further complicated by the variation in family patterns and their functional vs. dysfunctional potential depending on the sociocultural context and life cycle phase of each family (McGoldrick, Pearce, & Giordano, 1982; Carter & McGoldrick, 1980). Clinicians should avoid the error of labeling as pathological a family style that may be typical and functional in certain economic circumstances or ethnic contexts. Family systems evolve and interactional patterns change over time, both independent of and related to individual disorders. Labeling a family as a particular type, therefore, provides only a limited, cross-sectional view of the family at a particular point in time. One pattern may predominate — and even be functional — at one phase in a family's development, while the maintenance of the same pattern would be dysfunctional at another life stage. Arbitrary and unidimensional classification systems are too limited and simplistic to consider these multiple dimensions.

It is also important to recognize that the family patterns we see when a family member is in crisis or in the aftermath of a crisis may not reflect the family's prior style or optimal level of functioning. Under severe stress, a family system can change dramatically, appearing more dysfunctional as daily patterns are interrupted and unexpected challenges overwhelm family members and their ability to cope. However competent they might be at other times, under the stress which follows a suicide attempt, serious surgery, or psychotic break of a family member, almost all families would be likely to appear disorganized. As such families attempt to cope with chaos and restore their equilibrium, they are likely to become more rigid than usual in an effort to restore a sense of control and structure. They may develop unusual patterns or styles of interaction in attempts to avoid recurrent confrontations or to provide ongoing support to a vulnerable member. These patterns may appear inappropriate if compared to "normal" family standards, but be crucial to the survival of seriously ill individuals and their families during a crisis.

Just as there is a range of functioning among nonclinical families (Walsh, 1982; Lewis, Beavers, Gossett, & Phillips, 1976), families of disturbed patients vary in their functioning. In addition, some families cope well with certain aspects of the illness while other families cope poorly with these same symptoms. How well a family copes probably depends on a number of variables within the family system and in relationship to its social context (see Rolland, this volume). While the particular patterns of families with severely dysfunctional patients may vary, a common characteristic of those who cope less well is the tendency to be stuck in a particular mode of coping that doesn't work without being able to shift to another, more adaptive pattern. Future research should be attempted to identify variables, including systemic patterns, which enable families to cope effectively and maximize individual and family well-being.

FAMILY RESEARCH

To date, studies of families and severe disorders have generally been focused on a particular individual diagnosis, with most attention directed to schizophrenia (see Walsh in this volume), attempting to identify interactional patterns associated with the illness. Even more recent empirical research has, for the most part, been directed toward finding significant differences between families of patients in one diagnostic category and those in other categories. In fact, the finding of a family pattern is unlikely to be considered noteworthy — or publishable — if it is not linked exclusively to a particular disorder or found to differentiate the "study group" from "control groups." This emphasis on specificity leaves us with a set of problems. First, important variables may be overlooked that have a general, nonspecific disabling impact on vulnerable individuals and their families. Severe family stress, such as traumatic loss (see Walsh in this volume; Walsh & McGoldrick, 1987), may generate family disequilibrium that in interaction with other influences, may manifest itself in a variety of symptoms. The particular member who becomes most symptomatic and the form, severity and chronicity of dysfunction may vary with such factors as the biological predisposition of individual members, the confluence of other concurrent or past stresses, and family coping strategies and resources.

Second, the impact of *any* severe, chronic illness on family members may be more significant than the differences in impact between two disorders. Commonalities across diagnoses in such areas as problem-solving, stress management, and coping tend to be overlooked because they are statistically insignificant in differentiating diagnostic groups, and are therefore deemed unimportant in understanding a particular disorder. Such data analysis and research design practices reflect the bias that continues to permeate the clinical field: interest in the family is chiefly in its presumed causal role in the development or maintenance of major disorders. In considering such data "non-findings," important information is lost that may have considerable clinical value.

It is a misapplication of systems theory to view all individual problems as stemming from the family system or to presume that any family dysfunction present necessarily caused or maintains individual dysfunction. A true systems perspective requires recognition of the reciprocal influences of the individual, family and other systems. While patient behavior is embedded in family transactional processes, it generates stress on the family system just as it is responsive to stress. In schizophrenia for instance, the natural upset that family members feel because of illness, added to the ongoing intensity of family relationships, may create an emotional climate that escalated the patient's distress, producing increasingly disturbed behavior, which in turn generates more distress in family interactions in upwardly spiraling sequences. Moreover, clinicians should be cautioned not to presume that the disturbed behavior of an individual necessarily serves a function for the family. A family may be coping as well as could be expected given the constraints reality imposes on the family, and the limitations imposed by a particular disorder. More recent schizophrenia research has shifted away from etiological questions and causal inferences, attending instead to ongoing family influences that contribute to the course and treatment of the disorder. Major findings regarding the influence of communication processes, in particular, "expressed emotion," in the course and treatment of chronic schizophrenia are now being extended to other severe disorders, such as depression (Hooley, 1985). Whereas psychiatric research to date has concentrated on dysfunctional attributes of families, recent investigations of well functioning families also have increased our awareness that family strengths must be identified and promoted. How some families learn to cope effectively with biologically-based deficits in a member must be understood in order to develop intervention programs to help those who manage less well.

Even if presenting family patterns are largely reactive to the stress of coping with a disorder or with the stigma of hospitalization, they yield important information about the ways in which these factors may be traumatic for families or produce other stress related problems. Reactive dysfunctions must be identified and respected if clinicians are to be responsive to family distress. Treatment programs must address the experience and needs of families as well as patients if we are to alter patterns set in motion by either the disorder itself or hospital and previous treatment experiences. Without intervention, these patterns may affect the course of the illness negatively, lessening prospects for optimal functioning of both patients and their families.

In sum, empirical research models and methods of analysis have largely tended to reinforce a fragmented view and have failed to "capture" the reciprocity of individual and family influences in the development, course and treatment of chronic illness. While a few adherents of family systems theory have rejected empirical investigation on the basis that it is not systemic (Tomm, 1983), we would argue, along with others (Gurman, Kniskern, & Pinsof, 1986) that the baby should not be tossed out with the bath water. The problem, in large part, is not existing methodology but our lack of skill and specificity in applying it. What is needed is more refined conceptualization of hypotheses and variables and more sophisticated designs. For example, current methodological guidelines do not preclude the recognition of the influence of the investigator and the research context, or a shift from simplistic linear associations of so-called discrete "independent" and "dependent" variables to complex multivariate analyses that more closely approximate life experience. Recent advances in research on patient and family influences in the course and treatment of schizophrenia, with extension to other severe disorders, provide useful models for future research efforts.

FAMILY INTERVENTION APPROACHES

There is an increasing awareness of the need to commit resources to the problems of families with chronically ill members, be the illness medical or psychiatric. The impact of illness, the stress of caregiving roles, combined with preexisting and/or concurrent stresses all should be addressed in designing clinical care for patients and families. Minimally, family intervention priorities should include: (1) reduction of the stressful impact of chronic disorders on the family; (2) provision of information about the medical/psychiatric condition, patient abilities and limitations, and prognosis; (3) concrete guidelines for stress reduction and problem-solving; and (4) linkage to supplementary services to support the efforts of families to maintain their patient members in the community.

Which family therapy models might most effectively address these needs is an open question. We lack controlled studies comparing different family intervention approaches with particular diagnostic groups, or with severe and chronic disorders in general. Proponents of various family therapy models—in particular, the strategic approach of Haley (1976) and Madanes (1984), and systemic therapy developed by the Milan Associates (Selvini Palazzoli, 1978; Selvini Palazzoli, Boscolo, Cecchin, & Prata, 1978)—contend that their approaches are effective with a range of severe disorders. However, evidence in support of those claims is meager since most of these approaches have not been studied using controlled clinical trials and adequate methodology (Gurman, Kniskern, & Pinsof, 1986; Anderson, 1986).

Several behavioral and psychoeducational family treatment interventions have demonstrated some efficacy, particularly when used in combination with psychotropic medication and social skills training (Anderson et al., 1980, 1986; Falloon et al., 1982; Goldstein et al., 1978; Goldstein & Kopeiken, 1981; Hogarty et al., 1986; Leff et al., 1985). These studies include documented evidence that the interventions used delay relapse, reduce family stress, and improve functioning for schizophrenic patients and their families. Similar approaches also show some promise in the treatment of severe affective disorders, although the evidence is minimal (Anderson et al., 1986). A number of projects are beginning to apply similar principles of intervention in chronic medical disorders.

It may be important to recognize the need for combined intervention strategies in the treatment of severe and chronic disorders. When problems have biochemical components that can be treated, as in schizophrenia, manic-depressive illness, and other affective disorders, long-term drug maintenance may be necessary to control the severity of symptoms and to prevent lengthy and repeated hospitalizations. For instance, family therapy combined with drug therapy has been found to be more effective than either intervention alone in preventing relapse in schizophrenia (Goldstein & Kopeikin, 1981; Hogarty, Anderson, & Reiss, et al., 1986). In the treatment of chemical dependence, most experts agree that family therapy must be combined with individual treatment of the drug or alcohol abuse if progress is to be made and maintained (see Schwartzman in this volume). In conjunction with family therapy, socialization groups may also be highly beneficial for patients with deficits in interpersonal functioning.

As Gurman and Kniskern (1981) stated in a review of family therapy outcome studies, the task for the 1980s is to determine what are (1) the elements of psychotherapy that fit with (2) particular elements of family functioning that become (3) the focus for intervention and change and that lead to (4) successful outcomes in therapy. With severe and chronic disorders, family therapy can take different forms and functions including family consultation and advocacy (Wynne, McDaniel, & Weber, 1986).

Crisis intervention should be made available to families in times of acute distress. Since most chronic, severe disorders involve periodic exacerbation of symptoms, it is vital that therapists maintain an immediate availability and an up-to-date knowledge of existing resources. Because each situation differs, clinicians attempting to help these families must be flexible in providing different interventions and responding to different family members as needs arise. At the same time, therapists must be able to be active and to provide enough structure to help temporarily disorganized and overwhelmed family members to gain perspective and control of frightening situations.

Patients with severe/chronic disorders may lack motivation for treatment, or even strongly resist it at a time when they need it most, i.e., when their behavior poses a serious threat to themselves or others. Clinicians, therefore, must be prepared to help families to involve patients in treatment or help family members to develop their own abilities to cope with acute episodes in ways that reduce stress to manageable proportions. Contracting with families during a crisis to use the post-crisis period to anticipate and prevent future crises is often crucial. Without such guidance, many families may rebound from one crisis to the next, achieving few gains over time except increased emotional exhaustion and eventual burnout.

Brief, problem-focused family therapy may be of use to many families with a range of severe and chronic disorders, particularly for those families who have given up hoping for change and who may need a dramatically new way of seeing an old problem. A number of family therapists have attempted to apply a combined structural and strategic intervention to this population. Indirect techniques, such as paradoxical interventions which reframe the family dilemma, are employed to help families to break nonproductive rigid interactional patterns or perspectives. With severe and chronic disorders, in which the degree of deficit is great and problems are longstanding, resolution of the presenting problem or "cure" may not be a realistic therapeutic goal. However, improved functioning and reduction of stress and conflict in family relationships can be achieved by setting clear, concrete, attainable objectives likely to be met during short-term contracts. Gains can then be sustained and setbacks averted in long-term monthly maintenance sessions, in multiple family therapy groups or self-help organizations.

Multiple family groups are particularly relevant with these populations since they can provide a vital network function for families who have common problems, who have been isolated, or who have been stigmatized by the patient's chronic problems (Anderson, 1982; Anderson et al., 1980; Steinglass et al., 1982; Strelnick, 1977; Zarit & Zarit, 1982). Multiple family groups during inpatient hospitalizations as well as during the post-hospital phase of illness give patients, parents, siblings, and spouses the opportunity to share similar experiences, provide mutual ongoing support, and expand one another's repertoire for crisis management and reduction of stress and conflict. These same goals can, and often are, addressed in self-help groups which provide support and information along with the opportunity to perform a helping role in relation to similar families struggling with similar problems. Members of these groups can provide a kind of assistance that cannot be obtained from even the most talented and understanding professionals, who by and large have not experienced living twenty-four hours a day over a period of years with severe and often life-threatening problems. Furthermore, these groups can develop valuable advocacy functions to increase the contributions of local, state, and federal resources. Adult daycare for patients and their families is another option to partially relieve family burden.

SUMMARY

The field is experiencing the development of new approaches to families of patients with chronic disorders. While the ultimate goal may be a more integrated biological family approach, the first step in this process for family-oriented researchers and clinicians must involve the identification of relevant family issues within and across specific disorders, be they medical or psychiatric. This process will lay the groundwork for a more collaborative relationship with biologically-oriented clinicians and researchers. The identification of family issues, in a way that does not unnecessarily pathologize families will also further the development of a more respectful, collaborative, and helpful relationship with families. If family-oriented professionals can appreciate what it means for families to have a family member develop serious and long-term dysfunction, and how difficult it is for families to cope over time, especially when they shoulder the burden of primary caregiving, it may increase the likelihood of genuine collaboration and the development of effective interventions that promote the well-being and enhanced functioning of both patients and families.

The following papers include a variety of approaches to the identification of family issues in severe and chronic disorders. The emphasis in each section differs, with some authors emphasizing family issues, others taking a more biological view. The authors, and in fact, the editors, may not agree completely with one anothers' conclusions about the meaning and significance of the issues discussed. We differ in our conceptualization of the issues and in our ideas as to what should be done about them. This in no way should diminish the importance of stating our current knowledge and arguing for our points of view. Not only is there room for disagreement, but this disagreement, freely expressed, should contribute to the development of more sophisticated concepts, greater integration of diverse knowledge, and more effective intervention strategies.

Regardless of the approach each of us takes to families with chronic disorders, however, the editors believe it is imperative to avoid two common pitfalls in this area of work: (1) the tendency to overpathologize families who are struggling with impossibly stressful situations; and (2) the danger of contributing to the ongoing polarization of the already divergent positions of medically- and family-oriented clinicians, as well as the polarization between professionals and family advocacy groups. For patients and families to benefit in the long run, collaboration is crucial.

REFERENCES

Anderson, C. M. (1986). The all-too-short trip from positive to negative connotation. *Journal of Marital and Family Therapy, 12*(4), 351-354.

Anderson, C. M. (1982). The community connection: The impact of social networks on family and individual functioning. In F. Walsh (Ed.), *Normal Family Processes*. New York: Guilford Press, 425-445.

Anderson, C. M., Griffin, S., Rossi, A., Pagonis, I., Holder, D. & Treiber, R. (1986). A comparative study of the impact of education vs. process groups for families of patients with affective disorders. *Family Process, 25*, 185-205.

Anderson, C. M., Hogarty, G. & Reiss, D. J. (1980). Family treatment of adult schizophrenic patients: A psychoeducational approach. *Schizophrenia Bulletin, 6*, 490-505.

Anderson, C. M., Reiss, D. J. & Hogarty, G. (1986). *Schizophrenia and the family*. New York: Guilford Press.

Carter, E. & McGoldrick, M. (Eds.). (1980). *The family life cycle: Framework for family therapy*. New York: Gardner Press.

Falloon, I. R. H., Boyd, J. L., McGill, C. W., Razoni, J., Moss, H. B. & Gilderman, H. A. (1982). Family management in the prevention of exacerbations of schizophrenia. *New England Journal of Medicine, 306*, 1437-1444.

Goldstein, M. J. & Kopeikin, H. (1981). Short and long term effects of combining drug and family therapy. In M. J. Goldstein (Ed.), *New developments in interventions with families of schizophrenics*. San Francisco: Jossey-Bass.

Goldstein, M. J., Rodnick, E. H., Evans, J. R., May, P. R. & Steinberg, M. (1978). Drug and family therapy in the aftercare of acute schizophrenia. *Archives of General Psychiatry, 35*, 1169-1177.

Gurman, A. & Kniskern, D. (1978). Research on marital and family therapy: Progress, perspective, and prospect. In S. Garfield & A. Bergin (Eds.), *Handbook of psychotherapy and behavior change*. (2nd ed.). New York: Wiley & Sons.

Gurman, A., Kniskern, D. & Pinsof, W. (1986). Research on the process and outcome of marital and family therapy. In S. Garfield & A. Bergin (eds.) *Handbook of psychotherapy and behavior change*. (3rd ed.). New York: Wiley & Sons.

Haley, J. (1976). *Problem-solving therapy*. San Francisco: Jossey-Bass.

Hogarty, G. E., Anderson, C. M., Reiss, D.J. et al. (1986). Family psychoeducation, social skills training and maintenance chemotherapy in the aftercare treatment of schizophrenia. *Archives of General Psychiatry, 43*, 633-642.

Hooley, J. M. (1985). Expressed emotion: A review of the critical literature. *Clinical Psychology Review, 5*, 119-139.

Lansky, M. (1981). *Family therapy and major psychopathology*. New York: Gwine & Stratton.

Leff, J., Kuipers, L., Berkowitz, R. & Sturgeon, D. (1985). A controlled trial of social intervention in the families of schizophrenic patients: Two year follow-up. *British Journal of Psychiatry, 146*, 594-600.

Lewis, J., Beavers, W. R., Gossett, J. & Phillips, V. (1976). *No single thread: Psychological health in family systems*. New York: Brunner/Mazel.

Madanes, C. (1984). *Behind the one-way mirror: Advances in the practice of strategic therapy*. San Francisco: Jossey-Bass.

McGoldrick, M., Pearce, J. & Giordano, J. (1982). *Ethnicity and family therapy*. New York: Guilford Press.

Olson, D. & Walsh, F. (in press). The circumplex model in clinical assessment and treatment. *Journal of Psychotherapy & the Family*, 4.

Russell, C., Olson, D., Sprenkle, D. & Atilano, R. (1983). From family symptom to family system: Review of family therapy research. *American Journal of Family Therapy*, 11, 3-14.

Selvini Palazzoli, M. (1978). *Self starvation. From individual to family therapy*. New York: Jason Aronson.

Selvini Palazzoli, M. (1986). Towards a general model of psychotic family games. *Journal of Marital & Family Therapy*, 12, 339-349.

Selvini Palazzoli, M., Boscolo, L., Cecchin, G. & Prata, G. (1978). *Paradox and counterparadox: Families in schizophrenic transaction*. New York: Jason Aronson.

Steinglass, P., Gonzalez, B. A., Doscovitz, I. & Teiss, D. (1982). Discussion groups for chronic hemodialysis patients and their families. *General Hospital Psychiatry*, 4, 7-14.

Strelnick, A. H. (1977). Multiple family group therapy: A review of the literature. *Family Process*, 16, 307-333.

Teece, J. J. & Cole, J. O. (1976). The distraction-arousal hypothesis, CNV, and schizophrenia. In D. I. Mostofsky (Ed.), *Behavior control and modification of physiological activity*. Englewood Cliffs, N.J.: Prentice-Hall, Inc.

Tomm, K. (1983). The old hat doesn't fit. *Family Therapy Networker*, 7, 39-41.

Walsh, F. (1982). Conceptualizations of normal family functioning. In F. Walsh (Ed.), *Normal family processes*. New York: Guilford Press.

Walsh, F. (1987). The clinical utility of normal family research. *Psychotherapy*.

Walsh, F. (in press). Treating severely dysfunctional families. New York: Guilford Press.

Walsh, F. & McGoldrick, M. (1987). Loss and the family life cycle. In C. Falicov (Ed.), *Family transitions: Continuity and change*. New York: Guilford Press.

Wynne, L., McDaniel, S. & Weber, T. (1986). *Systems consultation: A new perspective for family therapy*. New York: Guilford Press.

Zarit, J. M. & Zarit, S. H. (1982). Families Under Stress: Interventions for caregivers of senile dementia patients. *Psychotherapy: Theory, Research & Practice*, 19, 461-471.

Zubin, J. & Spring, B. (1977). Vulnerability: A new view of schizophrenia. *Journal of Abnormal Psychology*, 86, 103-126.

New Perspectives
on Schizophrenia
and Families

Froma Walsh

Instead of considering patients with the diagnosis dementia
praecox as having a disorder, I prefer to think of them as belong-
ing to a Greek letter society, the conditions for admission to
which are obscure, inclusion in and exclusion from the fraternity
are determined by considerations which vary from year to year,
and from place to place, and the directing board is not known.

MacFie Campbell, 1935

The diagnosis of schizophrenia accounts for over half of the mentally ill patients in over half of all hospital beds in this country alone.
A profoundly distressing disorder affecting thought, perception, affect, behavior, and relationships, schizophrenia has confounded researchers and clinicians in attempts to understand and treat it. The
precise nature, operation, and interaction of factors in the development of the disorder have remained obscure. However, recent advances have been made in our knowledge about biochemical and family influences in the course and treatment of schizophrenia. This paper
will examine these developments and their implications for clinical
practice.

Attempts to understand the transmission of schizophrenia have been
plagued by simplistic either/or arguments for genetic versus environmental explanations. This tendency has fostered a controversy over
whether any disturbance found in families of schizophrenic patients at
hospitalization is either causal *or* reactive to an individual member's
disorder. At one extreme are those who maintain that biology is destiny, and that any disturbances in family transactions are merely re-

Froma Walsh, PhD, is Associate Professor, University of Chicago.

sponses to the patient's illness. At the other extreme are those who argue that schizophrenia is merely a myth or a metaphor: that the "real" problem is the family (for society) that has caused—or needs to maintain—the symptomatic behavior. Biological determinists tend to rely on psychopharmacological intervention and too often fail to attend to family distress or to see any value in family involvement in treatment. Some family therapists have swung to the other end of the pendulum, focusing exclusively on intrafamilial processes and arguing vehemently against any labeling of illness, use of the diagnosis of schizophrenia, hospitalization, or medication (Haley, 1980). Such extreme positions imply an erroneous assumption of linear causality that has not been borne out in empirical research and that is inconsistent with an understanding of the spiraling of influences in the functioning of human systems. A true systems perspective must take into account the ongoing interaction of biological, psychological, family, and larger social systems.

Although the precise biochemical mechanisms involved in the development of schizophrenia are not as yet fully understood, there is considerable evidence for a psychophysiological dysfunction, involving a heightened sensitivity to environmental stimuli and a cognitive deficit in information processing (Dawson & Nuechterlein, 1985; Neuchterlein & Dawson, 1984). Yet it remains unclear to what extent this deficit arises from a genetic predisposition and to what extent it is a manifestation of biochemical changes produced by severe or chronic environmental stress. In clinical intervention, antipsychotic medication has clearly been demonstrated to be effective in regulating the extremes of arousal and focusing attention. No drugs, however, have been found to be effective in addressing the wide range of problems these individuals have in work, family, and social functioning. As recent studies, to be described below, have indicated, treatment programs that combine psychotropic medication, family, and social interventions have proved to be more effective than any single intervention in forestalling relapse and improving the functioning of schizophrenic patients in the community.

Thus, a general systems perspective is required to take into account the complex transactional processes whereby a vulnerable individual and family reciprocally influence each other in an ongoing pattern of mutual reinforcement. The scientific task is to learn in what ways the *transactional processes* that occur between patient and family contribute to and reinforce, through action *and* reaction, the course of a schizophrenic disorder and the well-being of the family.

While descriptive studies of ongoing family patterns and recollections of past relationships cannot directly answer etiological questions regarding the possible role of the family in the development of schizophrenia, such investigation is essential for identification and refinement of key hypotheses, variables, and methods for testing in subsequent longitudinal research. Furthermore, beyond questions of origin, it is important to study current family perceptions and functioning to understand the social context in which schizophrenia is embedded. In particular, we need to learn how the patient and family view their shared experience and pattern their interactions as they attempt to cope with stress. Regardless of origin, it is important to specify the ways in which the patient is embroiled in transactional processes that are associated with his/her irrational thinking, destructive behavior, and inappropriate relating, and that impede efforts at reintegration and more autonomous functioning. It is of prognostic and therapeutic value to identify dysfunctional family processes—even if they may be largely reactive to the disorder—so that intervention can be targeted to strengthen those particular components of family interaction for stress reduction and optimal patient and family functioning (Anderson, Reiss, & Hogarty, 1986; Walsh, in press; Walsh & Olson, in press).

Furthermore, knowledge about healthy family functioning can inform treatment approaches to strengthen those aspects of family functioning that will maximize the likelihood of good outcome in patient functioning (Walsh, 1982, 1987b, in press). Beyond patient functioning, knowledge of transactional processes related to the course of the disorder can also guide intervention designed to reduce family stress and caregiving burden and to provide useful guidelines in restructuring daily interaction in chronic cases requiring long-term care.

FROM "SCHIZOPHRENOGENIC MOTHER"

Associations between a number of family patterns and schizophrenia have been postulated by clinical theorists and investigators. The psychoanalytic tradition generated numerous parental studies through the 1950s. Because schizophrenia was the most severe and chronic disorder, it was assumed that its origin must lie in the earliest phases of development. Therefore, research and clinical attention focused narrowly on examination of mothering patterns in early childhood. This line of investigation was based on the linear causal assumption that maternal character deficiencies produced destructive patterns of mothering responsible for the child's disorder. The widely used concept of "schizophrenogenic mother," originated by Fromm-Reichmann (1948), was never consistently defined or measured and became a pejorative label that blamed mothers for causing schizophrenia, through their character deficiencies and "bad mothering" styles. Only a few impressionistic studies explored the possible contribution of fathers in schizophrenia, reporting them to be inadequate, passive, and peripheral (Alanen, 1966). Prevalent, throughout the field, was the value judgement that the father's only shortcoming was an "error of omission," in failing to uphold the dominant leadership role in the family thought to be essential for the healthy development of offspring (Lidz, et al., 1965) and necessary to control or counteract the mother's destructive behavior, or "errors of commission." Family assessments were, in effect, historical inquiries to uncover the failings of the parents. Because the field of mental health was so exclusively concerned with psychopathology, all attention to the family focused on presumed pathogenesis.

In the late 1950s a new level of conceptualization, observation, and analysis of the whole family as an interactional system was developed. While the aim of research on schizophrenia was still to understand the role of the family in the development of the disorder, the importance of ongoing transactional processes and an assumption of circularity of influences—including behavior of the schizophrenic member—replaced the deterministic stance of earlier models. Pioneering investigations were conducted by the Bateson group (1956) at the Mental Research Institute in Palo Alto; by Lidz and his Yale colleagues (1985); and at NIMH by Wynne and Singer (Wynne et al., 1958; Wynne & Singer, 1963a, 1963b; Singer & Wynne, 1965), and by Bowen (1960). Using a variety of methods to study whole families, these studies reported severe transactional disorders in family structure, communicational processes, and relational dynamics. (Readers are referred to the excellent review of early family research in schizophrenia by Mishler & Waxler, 1968.)

With few exceptions, early family studies in schizophrenia had serious methodological weaknesses, (as reviewed by Riskin & Faunce, 1972; Jacob, 1975.Conclusions were limited by small sample size; lack of nonschizophrenic disturbed or normal control groups; failure to control or test for the influences of such variables as social class, gender, and premorbid status; failure to operationalize constructs, procedures, and units of analysis; and questions of reliability and inference from impressionistic, informal clinical observation. Nevertheless, these studies were an important catalyst in the rapid development of the field of family therapy and they opened new territory for more systematic investigations of family processes in schizophrenia that followed.

Communication Deviance

One of the most notable research advances has been the line of systematic investigation of communication disorders, following the research strategy developed by Wynne and Singer (1963a, 1963b; Singer & Wynne, 1965). Initially, they used verbatim Rorschach and TAT protocols as a standardized procedure to measure communication *process*. Manuals were developed for scoring "communication deviances" (CD), assessed by their transactional impact on the listener (Singer & Wynne, 1966). CD categories include features of amorphous and fragmented communication, such as ambiguous and inconsistent references, disqualifications, and nihilistic and distracting remarks. In families of schizophrenic patients, communication was found to be disturbed in the basic sharing of a focus of attention, leading to failures in sharing meaning, in establishing appropriate closeness/distance, and in acquiring a sense of trust in the family's relational reality. A large body of research has corroborated and extended this work, finding a consistent relationship between parental communication deviance (CD) and the diagnosis of schizophrenia or schizophreniform disorders in offspring (Wynne, Singer, Bartko, & Toohey, 1977; Wild, Shapiro, & Goldenberg, 1974; Jones, 1977; Doane, West, Goldstein, Rodnick, & Jones, 1981; Tienari, 1984).

Expressed Emotion

The work of Brown and his colleagues (Brown, Birley, & Wing, 1972), followed by the investigations of Vaughn and Leff (1976a, 1976b) found empirical evidence linking the course of the schizophrenic disorder with certain attitudes expressed by family members about the patient, presumably reflecting ongoing family transactions. The concept of expressed emotion (EE) refers to "an index of familial attitudes shown to be a powerful predictor of schizophrenic relapse" by the patient (Leff & Vaughn, 1985). More specifically, critical comments and emotional overinvolvement have been identified as most highly predictive of later symptomatic relapse by the patient. Findings of relapse associated with high expressed emotion by spouses and other relatives besides parents suggests that current interaction — not simply long-term development — is crucial in the course of the illness and can be an important focus for intervention.

While EE is a rating of family member attitudes based on a structured individual interview about the patient, a related concept of affective style (AS), developed by Doane and her associates (Doane, West, Goldstein, Rodnick, & Jones, 1981; Doane, Falloon, Goldstein, & Mintz, 1985) measures actual emotional behavior observed during direct interaction of family members, including the patient. The AS scoring system includes ratings of benign and personal criticism, guilt induction, and critical and neutral intrusiveness. When EE and AS have been rated on the same sample, high parental EE scores were found to correlate with more negative AS in direct interaction. When studied in combination with parental communication deviance, family affective style has also been found to predict disturbed versus benign long-term outcome of vulnerable adolescents (Doane et al., 1981; Goldstein & Doane, 1982). Wynne (1984) has proposed an epigenetic model of family development, suggesting that EE and AS are associated with the attachment/caregiving phase of relational development, while CD is more relevant to the development of communication processes involving attentional sharing, cognitive functioning, and language development.

Of note when considering schizophrenia in comparison to other severe and chronic disorders, EE patterns have been found to be nonspecific for schizophrenia. A comparison group of depressive patients was found to be even more sensitive to criticism, which strongly predicted relapse of depression (Vaughn & Leff, 1976; Hooley et al., 1986). High expressed emotion has also been found to predict the course of anorexia nervosa and of weight-maintenance in obese women (Leff & Vaughn, 1985). Such reports underscore the need for further study on these and other measures of family communication for individuals with a range of severe and chronic disorders. In delineating specific aspects of a family transaction that can influence the course of a disorder, we improve our ability to target family intervention to alter those particular patterns to strengthen patient and family functioning.

Other aspects of family interaction were investigated by Walsh and colleagues (Walsh, 1987a; Grinker & Holzman, 1973) through systematic assessment of interviews and questionnaires, projective story construction, and structured conjoint task. Young adult schizophrenic patients were found to differ significantly from demographically comparable nonschizophrenic hospitalized and normal control groups on several family relational variables. In family structure, triadic relationships with parents were distinguished by a breaching of generational boundaries in perceptions and communication of triangulated mate-like distortions of parent-child relationships (Walsh, 1979). An assessment of patient, parents, and sibling perceptions of dyadic relation-ships (Summers & Walsh 1977, 1979, 1980, 1981) found that: (1) the relationship between the schizophrenic patient and mother was per-ceived by all family members as poorly differentiated, with separation concerns for the mother's well-being as much as for the schizophrenic patient; (2) fathers were viewed as lacking in confirmation (acknowl-edgment and accommodation) toward the patient; (3) parents' marital relationships showed similar patterns, with perceptions of undifferen-tiation and overdependency on husbands by mothers and lack of con-firmation of their wives by fathers; and (4) intergenerational patterns with the schizophrenic patient were not found for sibling-parent rela-tionships. An investigation of family stress and developmental transi-tions (Walsh, 1978) found a significantly higher concurrence of grand-parent death with the birth of the schizophrenic offspring (41%) than with nonschizophrenic patients (20%) or normal offspring (8%). Indi-cations of persistent unresolved mourning suggested that in many fam-ilies, the patient may assume a replacement function, complicating later separation attempts. Similar patterns were reported by McGoldrick (in Walsh, 1978; Mueller & McGoldrick Orfanidis, 1976). Other researchers (Coleman & Stanton, 1978; Coleman, 1986) have found traumatic loss in families of severe drug abusers linked to separation difficulties and self-destructive behavior by the addict. Such findings point to the need for further research on the confluence of different family patterns of adaptation to loss with varying patient vulnerabilities in a range of severe disorders (Walsh & McGoldrick, 1987; Walsh, McGoldrick, & Rohrbaugh, in preparation).

In sum, more recent empirical studies to date have assumed the mutual, ongoing influence of biological and environmental factors in the development and course of schizophrenia. Family relational attrib-utes reported and observed at the time of patient hospitalization must be considered at least in part reactive to the schizophrenic disorder, since ongoing transactions both shape and are shaped by the vulnera-bilities and deficits of an individual family member. Research focus has shifted away from the backward search for origin to primary con-cern about future course and intervention foci to influence outcome. The work on communication deviance, expressed emotion, and affec-tive style provide the strongest evidence that family evaluations at the time of a psychotic episode can provide valuable prognostic informa-tion about the likelihood of relapse and can offer guidelines for effec-tive family intervention targeted to modify dysfunctional transactional processes.

RECENT DEVELOPMENTS IN FAMILY INTERVENTION

With the deinstitutionalization movement and the need to provide community based services for schizophrenic patients and their families, clinicians have been increasingly involved in family intervention. However, the severity and chronicity of problems present challenges to even seasoned therapists who find traditional intervention approaches to be inappropriate and ineffective. Too often, families with a schizophrenic member have experienced family therapy as yet another treatment context in which they have felt blamed by overt or covert implications that they have been responsible for causing or for maintaining the individual's disorder (Hatfield & Lefly, in press). Given the research findings of heightened levels of criticism and sensitivity to it in families of schizophrenics, therapists need to be more attuned to the impact of family assessments focused primarily on negative attributes, i.e., discovering faulty parenting patterns. Interventions pointing out observed parental failures in communication or problem-solving tend only to make families feel more inadequate and guilty. It is not surprising that families, who in previous experience with mental health professionals have been regarded as noxious influences, may become defensive and drop out of treatment in reaction to—or expectation of—attribution of blame. Such response is, then, too often simply viewed as resistance "in" the family or the family is dismissed as untreatable.

Structural-Strategic and Systemic Approaches

Structural-strategic and systemic approaches to family intervention have been reported to be highly effective in treating a range of problems, including schizophrenia, although there is little empirical evidence, to date, to support claims of the efficacy of these models with schizophrenia (Gurman, Kniskern & Pinsof, 1986; Selvini Palazzoli, 1986; Anderson, 1986). These models have emphasized the use of indirect methods of change, including paradoxical intervention techniques, to modify rigid transactional patterns in which schizophrenic systems appear to be embedded (Haley, 1980; Selvini Palazzoli, Boscolo, Cecchin & Prata, 1978).

Many family therapists from a structural-strategic or systemic orientation have been adverse to the use of diagnostic labels, hospitalization, or medication, out of concern that they will reinforce a "patient" role. The Milan associates, in particular, have rightly underscored the importance of maintaining a neutral stance, of connoting positively the benign intentions of family members, and of employing circular questioning to correct erroneous linear views of the cause or nature of problems. However, therapists need to be cautious that a conflicting message connoting negative intentions and blame may be conveyed to families by an assumption that symptomatic behavior serves a function for a family; that members need to maintain the problem (to avoid other problems or feared consequences of change); that these families are like "barracudas" (Bergman, 1985); or that the family is "playing" "dirty games" (see Selvini Palazzoli, 1986; Anderson, 1986). A mutually destructive transactional process among family members — including the patient — may, in fact, have evolved over time in many cases. Nevertheless, to regard the patient as victim and other family members (in particular, the parents or the mother) as villains is neither accurate nor helpful. Given the historical context of attribution of blame to families, clinicians need to be careful even in use of the term "dysfunctional." The term should be used to mean only that interactional processes are not working well and that individual members and/or the family as a unit are distressed; it should not be used to imply family origin or responsibility for that distress (Walsh, in press, and 1987b).

Psychoeducational Models

The most promising advance in family intervention with schizophrenia has been the development of psychoeducational models. In contrast to the models above, these are rather straightforward approaches that define schizophrenia as an illness, provide family education about the disorder, and offer concrete guidelines and support for crisis management, problem-solving, and stress reduction. These programs are also designed to provide crisis-oriented aftercare during the critical transition of reentry from the hospital to the community. In traditional treatment programs, too often there is a fragmentation between hospital treatment and aftercare in the community, with family support terminating or in transfer at hospital discharge, precisely the time that is most stressful, when the patient is at greatest risk of relapse, and when continuity of care is most essential. Moreover, when family therapy is recommended following hospitalization, too often the explicit or implicit rationale conveyed to the family is that family therapy is indicated *because* the family is pathological and destructive to the patient. In contrast, psychoeducational approaches engage the family as valued and essential collaborators in the treatment process, and explicitly base the rationale for family intervention on the importance of practical information, support, and problem-solving assistance through the predictably stressful transition period ahead that all patients and families must navigate.

Goldstein and his colleagues (Goldstein et al., 1978; Goldstein, 1981; Goldstein & Kopeikin, 1981) conducted the first controlled studies that demonstrated the combined effectiveness of drug and family therapy in preventing rehospitalization and reducing dysfunctional symptoms following hospital discharge of young first- and second-admission schizophrenic patients. The combination of family therapy and drug maintenance was found to be more effective than either family therapy or drugs alone in helping patients maintain functioning in the community during the high risk period following hospitalization. The Goldstein model of family therapy was brief (six weeks), problem-focused, and concrete. The aims of the program were to identify specific stressful events of current concern to the patient and family and then to help families develop coping strategies to prevent the recurrence of such events or to mitigate their destructive impact. Interactional conflicts and stresses viewed as potential precipitants of a psychotic episode were emphasized. When symptoms, per se, were labeled as stressors by family members, attempts were made to shift the focus to the interpersonal consequences of symptoms. Families were helped to develop and implement coping skills through direct teaching, coaching, and practice. When problems arose, obstacles to the implementation process were examined and coping strategies modified. Finally, patients and families were helped to anticipate and plan how they would handle future stress.

The psychoeducational model developed by Anderson and her colleagues (Anderson, Hogarty, & Reiss, 1980, 1981; Anderson, Reiss, & Hogarty, 1986) has most impressively demonstrated effectiveness in the treatment of chronic schizophrenia and reduction of family distress. Family intervention combined with drug maintenance and patient social skills training produced the best results with chronic patients, actually reducing the relapse rate to zero in the first year.

The intervention model is based on the assumption that the patient has a core biological deficit and that environmental sources of stress interact negatively with that deficit to produce disturbed cognitions and behaviors. Families are viewed as a resource for the long-term management of schizophrenia when given concrete support and information to assist them. A highly structured family-oriented program was designed to avoid treatment dropout, to decrease relapse rates, to return the patient to effective functioning in the community, and to decrease family stress. The basic goals of the program are: (1) decreased patient vulnerability to environmental stimulation through maintenance chemotherapy; and (2) increased stability and predictability of the family environment by decreasing family anxiety about the patient, increasing their knowledge about the schizophrenic illness, and increasing their confidence about their ability to manage it. As these aims are achieved, reciprocal pressures between the patient and the family are reduced.

The intervention program is operationalized in five phases. Phase I, connecting with the family, establishes an alliance with families by attending, in a noncritical manner, to the family's needs and experience and to specific areas of stress in their lives. Phase II is a day long survival skills workshop that provides a group of families with current empirically based knowledge about schizophrenia and its treatment, emphasizing the importance of medication compliance in avoiding relapse. Concrete principles and techniques for managing the illness are outlined, with information about what families can realistically expect. Families are encouraged to set clear limits on the patient's disruptive behavior and to shift attention and time to other family members' needs and to their own pursuits outside the family. Phase III involves ongoing supportive sessions, every two to three weeks for a year or two, based on themes from the workshop, in particular, reinforcement of family boundaries and gradual resumption of patient responsibilities. Phase IV, continued treatment or disengagement, offers families two options once patients are stabilized at what seems to be their optimal level of functioning and once basic contract goals have been reached. Families may elect traditional family therapy to resolve long-term conflicts, or else periodic supportive maintenance sessions. For patients who have been ill for many years, some ongoing supportive contact, however minimal, is recommended rather than complete termination, since periodic exacerbations of symptoms are likely.

Another psychoeducational model developed by Falloon and his colleagues (Falloon, Boyd, & McGill, 1984; Falloon et al., 1986) is a home based family intervention approach, emphasizing behavioral problem-solving techniques. Although home based intervention is generally considered to be too time consuming to be practical, Falloon has demonstrated that his model is actually more cost-effective than other approaches.

CONCLUSION

Many of the principles of the psychoeducational models have been combined with other approaches or adapted to fit different client needs and treatment settings in broad based clinical practice with a range of severe and chronic disorders (Bernheim & Lehman, 1985; Walsh, in press). McFarlane (1983) has developed a decision tree to assist clinicians in the determination and sequencing of treatment approaches and priorities in different case situations. Family consultation, a model recently advanced by Wynne and his colleagues (Wynne, McDaniel, & Weber, 1986) holds promise as an alternative to family therapy. Setting concrete, realistic objectives in active collaboration with families is a hallmark of all of these recent approaches.

This is a time of controversy and creative energy in the clinical field, with heated debates among proponents of different conceptual and practice models. Consumers — the families themselves — who have become quite vocal in their criticism of traditional approaches to individual and family treatment of schizophrenia, have been enthusiastic in their response to psychoeducational and other similar approaches. The emerging body of research yields evidence for cautious optimisim that, indeed, progress is being made in understanding and being helpful to schizophrenic patients and their families.

REFERENCES

Alanen, Y. O. et al., (1966). The family in the pathogenesis of schizophrenic and neurotic disorders. *Acta Psychiatrica Scandinavia*, *42*, Suppl. 189.

Anderson, C. M. (1986). The all-too-short trip from positive to negative connotation. *Journal of Marital & Family Therapy*, *12*, 351-354.

Anderson, C. M., Hogarty, G., & Reiss, D. (1980). Family treatment of adult schizophrenic patients: A psychoeducational approach. *Schizophrenia Bulletin*, *6*, 490-505.

Anderson, C. M., Hogarty, G., & Reiss, D. (1981). The psychoeducational family treatment of schizophrenia. In M. Goldstein (Ed.), *New developments in interventions with families of schizophrenics*. San Francisco: Jossey-Bass.

Anderson, C. M., Reiss, D., & Hogarty, G. (1986). *Schizophrenia and the Family*. New York: Guilford Press.

Bateson, G., Jackson, D., Haley, J., & Weakland, J. (1956). Toward a theory of schizophrenia. *Behavioral Science*, *1*, 251-264.

Bergman, J. (1985). *Fishing for barracuda*. New York: W.W. Norton.

Bernheim, K., & Lehman (1985). *Working with families of the mentally ill*. New York: W.W. Norton.

Bowen, M. (1960). A family concept of schizophrenia. In D. Jackson (Ed.), *The etiology of schizophrenia*. New York: Basic Books.

Brown, G. W., Birley, J. L. T., & Wing, J. K. (1972). Influence of family life on the course of schizophrenic disorders: A replication. *British Journal of Psychiatry*, *121*, 241-258.

Coleman, S., Kaplan, J., & Downing, R. (1986). Life cycle and loss — The spiritual vacuum of heroin addiction. *Family Process*, *25*, 5.

Coleman, S., & Stanton, D. (1978). The role of death in the addict family. *Journal of Marriage & Family Counseling*. *4*, 79-91.

Dawson, M., & Neuchterlein, K. (1985). Psychophysiological dysfunctions in the developmental course of schizophrenic disorders. *Schizophrenia Bulletin*, *10*, 204-232.

Doane, J., West, K., Goldstein, M., Rodnick, E., & Jones, J. (1981). Parental communication deviance and affective style: Predictors of subsequent schizophrenia spectrum disorders in vulnerable adolescents. *Archives of General Psychiatry*, *38*, 679-685.

Doane, J., Falloon, I., Goldstein, M., & Mintz, J. (1985). Parental affective style and the treatment of schizophrenia. *Archives of General Psychiatry, 42,* 34-46.

Falloon, I., Boyd, J., & McGill, C. (1984). *Family care of schizophrenia: A problem-solving approach to the treatment of mental illness.* New York: Guilford Press.

Fromm-Reichmann, F. (1948). Notes on the development of treatment of schizophrenia by psychoanalytic psychotherapy. *Psychiatry, 11,* 263-273.

Goldstein, M. (Ed.). (1981). *New developments in interventions with families of schizophrenics.* San Francisco: Jossey-Bass.

Goldstein, M., Rodnick, E., Evans, J., May, P., & Steinberg, M. (1978). Drug and family therapy in the aftercare treatment of acute schizophrenics. *Archives of General Psychiatry, 35,* 1169-1177.

Goldstein, M., & Doane, J. (1982). Family factors in the onset, course, and treatment of schizophrenic spectrum disorders: An update on current research. *Journal of Nervous and Mental Disease, 170,* 692-700.

Goldstein, M., & Kopeikin, H. (1981). Short- and long-term effects of combining drug and family therapy. In M. Goldstein (Ed.), *New developments in interventions with families of schizophrenics.* San Francisco: Jossey Bass.

Grinker, R., & Holzman, P. (1973). Schizophrenic pathology in young adults. *Archives of General Psychiatry, 28,* 168-175.

Gurman, A., Kniskern, D., & Pinsof, W. (1986). Research on the process and outcome of marital and family therapy. In S. Garfield & A. Bergin (Eds.), *Handbook of psychotherapy and behavior change.* (2nd ed.). New York: Wiley & Sons.

Haley, J. (1980). *Leaving home.* New York: McGraw-Hill.

Hatfield, A., & Lefley, H. (in press). *Families of the mentally ill: Coping and adaptation.* New York: Guilford Press.

Jacob, T. (1975). Family interaction in disturbed and normal families: A methodological and substantive review. *Psychological Bulletin, 38,* 35-65.

Jones, J. (1977). Patterns of transactional style deviance in the TAT's of parents of schizophrenics. *Family Process, 16,* 327-337.

Leff, J., & Vaughn, C. (1985). *Expressed emotion in families: Its significance for mental illness.* New York: Guilford Press.

Lidz, T., Fleck, S., & Cornelison, A. (1965). *Schizophrenia and the family.* New York: International Universities Press.

McFarlane, W. (Ed.). (1983). *Family therapy in schizophrenia.* New York: Guilford Press.

Mishler, E., & Waxler, N. (1968). Family interaction and schizophrenia. *Journal of Psychiatric Research, 6,* 213-222.

Mueller, P., & Orfanidis (McGoldrick), M. (1976). A method of co-therapy for schizophrenic families. *Family Process, 15,* 179-191.

Neuchterlein, K., & Dawson, M. (1984). Information processing and attentional functioning in the developmental course of schizophrenic disorders. *Schizophrenia Bulletin, 10,* 160-203.

Riskin, J., & Faunce, E. (1972). An evaluative review of family interaction research. *Family Process, 11,* 365-455.

Selvini Palazzoli, M. (1986). Towards a general model of psychotic family games. *Journal of Marital & Family Therapy, 12,* 339-349.

Selvini Palazzoli, M., Boscolo, L., Cecchin, G., & Prata, G. (1978). *Paradox and Counterparadox.* New York: Jason Aronson.

Singer, M. T., & Wynne, L. C. (1965). Thought disorder and family relations of schizophrenics. IV: Results and implications. *Archives of General Psychiatry, 12,* 201-212.

Singer, M. T., & Wynne, L. C. (1966). principles for scoring communication defects and deviances in parents of schizophrenics: Rorschach & TAT scoring manuals. *Psychiatry, 29,* 260-288.

Summers, F., & Walsh, F. (1977). The nature of the symbiotic bond between mother and schizophrenic. *American Journal of Orthopsychiatry, 47,* 484-494.

Summers, F., & Walsh, F. (1979). Symbiosis and confirmation between father and schizophrenic. American Journal of Orthopsychiatry, 49, 136-148.

Summers, F., & Walsh, F. (1980). Schizophrenic and sibling: A comparison of parental relationships. American Journal of Family Therapy, 8, 45-52.

Summers, F., & Walsh, F. (1981). Symbiosis and confirmation between the parents of the schizophrenic. Family Process, 20, 319-330.

Tienari, P. (1984). The Finnish adoptive family study of schizophrenics. Paper presented at VIIIth International Symposium on the Psychotherapy of Schizophrenia, Yale University, New Haven, CT.

Vaughn, C., & Leff, J. (1976). The measurement of expressed emotion in the families of psychiatric patients. British Journal of Social & Clinical Psychology, 15, 157-165.

Walsh, F. (1978). Concurrent grandparent death and birth of schizophrenic offspring: An intriguing finding. Family Process, 17, 457-463.

Walsh, F. (1979). Breaching of family generation boundaries by schizophrenics, disturbed, and normals. International Journal of Family Therapy, 1, 254-275.

Walsh, F. (1982). Conceptualizations of normal family functioning. In F. Walsh (Ed.), Normal family processes. New York: Guilford Press.

Walsh, F. (In press). Treating Severely Dysfunctional Families. New York: Guilford Press.

Walsh, F. (1987a). Family relationship patterns in schizophrenia. In R. R. Grinker & M. Harrow (Eds.), Clinical research in schizophrenia: A multidimensional approach. Springfield, IL: Thomas.

Walsh, F. (1987b). The clinical utility of normal family processes. Psychotherapy, 23, 3.

Walsh, F., & McGoldrick, M. (1987). Loss and the family life cycle. In C. Falicov (Ed.), Family transitions: Continuity and change. New York: Guilford Press.

Walsh, F., McGoldrick, M., & Rohrbaugh, M. (in preparation). Family adaptation to loss in schizophrenia, other severe disorders, and normal families.

Walsh, F., & Olson, D. H. (in press). The circumplex model in assessment and treatment of severely dysfunctional families. Journal of Psychotherapy & the Family, 4.

Wild, C., Shapiro, L., & Goldenberg, L. (1975). Transactional communication disturbances in families of male schizophrenics. Family Process, 14, 131-160.

Wynne, L.C. (1984). The epigenesis of relational systems: A model for understanding family development. Family Process, 23, 297-318.

Wynne, L. C., Rycoff, I., Day, J., & Hirsch, S. (1958). Pseudo-mutuality in the family relations of schizophrenics. Psychiatry 21, 205-220.

Wynne, L. C., & Singer, M. (1963a). Thought disorder and family relations of schizophrenics: I. A research strategy. Archives of General Psychiatry, 9, 191-198.

Wynne, L. C. & Singer, M. (1963b). Thought disorder and family relations of schizophrenics: II. A classification of forms of thinking. Archives of General Psychiatry, 9, 199-206.

Wynne, L. C.., Singer, M., Bartlo, J., & Toohey, M. (1977). Schizophrenics and their families: Recent research on parental communication. In J. M. Tanner (Ed.), Developments in psychiatric research. London: Hodder & Stoughton.

Depression and Families

Carol Anderson

Depression has many faces, not all of them characterized by sadness and tears. The young mother who cannot gather enough energy to care for her children, the middle-aged man who has lost interest in his career, the young child who is constantly irritable, all may be experiencing depression. In fact, millions of Americans suffer from depression, since it is *the* most common psychiatric disorder, affecting over 10% of the population. Approximately one in five women and one in nine men will experience a serious depressive episode sufficiently serious to cause them to seek treatment at some point in their lives. Of those who become severely depressed, 15% will experience these symptoms recurrently (Weissman & Akiskal, 1984). Many additional people will have chronic problems with their mood and self-esteem, will experience dysphoria or dysthymia without their symptoms becoming sufficiently severe that they can be labeled "depressed" using official DSM-III criteria (Spitzer, 1978). The toll of depression, however, is not limited to those who suffer from it directly. It also affects the families, friends and associates of those with the disorder. As Shervert Frazier, Director of the NIMH, has stated, "Just about everybody is related to someone who's suffering from depression" (Gallagher, 1986, p. 68). Thus, depression affects a staggering number of individuals, many with such a severe impact as to influence their ability to work or interact with those around them.

Depression and family issues are likely to be intertwined in many and complicated ways. Genetic, developmental, stress, and ongoing interactional factors are all thought to be relevant in the etiology, course and outcome of this serious mental health problem. There is evidence that those who later receive a diagnosis of depression often have problems related to their families of origin that begin in early

Carol Anderson, PhD, is Professor, Department of Psychiatry, University of Pittsburgh, and Director of the Family Institute of Pittsburgh.

Reprint requests may be addressed to Carol Anderson, PhD, Professor, Department of Psychiatry, University of Pittsburgh, 3811 Ohara Street, Pittsburgh, PA 15213.

childhood (Blatt et al., 1976; Parker, 1979; Perris, 1971; Lewine et al., 1978). In particular, the family histories of patients with characterologic and/or neurotic depressions seem to have a higher prevalence of alcohol and drug abuse, affective disorders (Andreason & Winokur, 1979) and early loss (Akiskal et al., 1978; Brown et al., 1977; Roy, 1981; Rosenthal et al., 1981; Merikangas et al., 1985).

Depressed adults are likely to suffer from chronically low self-esteem and hopelessness, problems in and of themselves, but also potentially powerful factors in the development of relationship problems (Eidelson & Epstein, 1982). While not all depressed individuals report marital problems (Hops et al., 1983) marital relationships of depressed patients do appear to be at increased risk. Depressed women, in fact, often present with marital problems as one of their primary complaints (Weissman et al., 1974; Bromet & Cornely, 1984). Both controlled and uncontrolled studies have attempted to speculate on the reasons for the high incidence of marital unhappiness in this population. Many suggest that a negative marital environment contributes to the etiology or onset of the disorder (Briscoe & Smith, 1973; Hinchliffe et al., 1975; Weissman, 1972). Variables which have been cited as contributing factors include the husband's dominance (Hoover & Fitzgerald, 1981; Collins et al., 1971) a lack of intimacy and autonomy (Weissman & Paykel, 1974), coercive relationships characterized by struggles for control (Seligman et al., 1979; McLean & Hakistan, 1979), generally "unsustaining environments," reduced general affective involvement or disengagement between partners (Bothwell & Weissman, 1977), unfulfilled role expectations, reduced affection and reduced reciprocity (Weissman & Paykel, 1974). In addition, families of depressed inpatients appear to have more disturbed communication and problem solving abilities than others, problems which were more striking when it was the mother in the family who was depressed (Kreitner et al., 1984).

Unfortunately, almost all studies of family variables and depression have serious methodological flaws. In particular, most of these studies rely on self-reports of already depressed individuals, failing to include either the reports of other family members or direct observations of family interaction. (See Kreitner et al., 1984, for a good review of these studies along with a critique of their methodology.) Thus it is impossible to conclude to what extent negative statements or judgements about their marital relationships were a reflection of a patient's depression, an individual's depressed state caused the marital distress, or marital problems contributed to the development of depression.

However, it seems clear to a large number of researchers and clinicians that lack of control is an important factor in the development and course of depression. In one of the few controlled studies of the marriages of depressed patients which was based on direct observations of patients and their spouses, Hinchcliffe and her colleagues (Hinchliffe et al., 1975; Hinchliffe et al., 1978) reported a number of relevant interpersonal factors in the marital interaction. They found the existence of negative, uneven, or overly protective interactions which lacked the support or the tension release of humor that was characteristic of control couples. In comparing couples in which one spouse was hospitalized for medical reasons with couples in which one spouse was hospitalized for depression, they found those in the depressed group to have significantly more tension, negative communication, disruption of each other's messages, self-preoccupation, and incongruence between nonverbal body movements and verbal communications (Hinchliffe et al., 1975). Surprisingly, depressed women actually made more verbal and nonverbal *attempts* to control their spouses than the comparison group, especially when they were acutely ill. They tended to speak more, interrupt more and use more eye gaze than did nondepressed wives, or than they themselves did after the acute episode subsided. Thus, it is possible that control itself is less important than the *perception* of control. Perhaps depressed women, rather than actually being dominated by their husbands, are more likely to *perceive* themselves as lacking control, are more dissatisfied with the amount of control they have, or the ineffectiveness of their efforts to control exacerbated their feelings of helplessness and depression.

While control is probably an important variable in intimate relationships, and may even be a contributing factor in the development of depression, the negative marital and family interactional sequences that arise from a depressed person's symptoms and requests for reassurance are probably also significant. For instance, if an individual has a tendency to feel worthless and helpless, he/she is likely to be oversensitive to any messages that are perceived to reinforce these feelings (McCranie, 1971). Thus (McCranie, 1971), depressed persons suffering from a diffuse misery may make excessive demands for reassurance from their families and may even dominate others with messages of blame or demands for emotional comfort (Bonine, 1960, 1966; Weissman & Paykel, 1974). Genuine reassurance may not be forthcoming, since the depressed person may be engaging others in a way that alienates them, thus, actually decreasing support and encouraging others to send more "depressing" information. This, in turn, would be likely to reinforce the depressed person's already existing self-doubt and low self-esteem (Cammer, 1971; Golin et al., 1981). Even when a spouse or other family member is able to give reassurance, the distorted view of the world inherent in depression may dominate information processing to the extent that the depressed individual does not receive or accept positive messages and information (Golin et al., 1981). In this way, interactive and cognitive factors may play important roles in exacerbating, maintaining or causing both depression and family conflict.

Depressed individuals do seem to be particularly sensitive to criticism, and some suggest that this in turn seems to have an impact on the course of the disorder. Studies of expressed emotion (EE) in relatives of depressed individuals, found them to be no more critical of patients than relatives of schizophrenic patients, but found that as few as two critical comments by a relative to be predictive of relapse (Vaughn & Leff, 1976). Others maintain there is no support for the hypothesis that criticism is central in the outcome of depressive disorders, at least as it relates to the husbands of depressed women (Goering et al., 1984).

Clearly, however, the negative interactional patterns that exist for many depressed individuals are not restricted to spouses and other intimates, but rather are a part of a more general response depressed individuals elicit from their social environments. In a study in which women students engaged in a telephone conversation with either a depressed patient, a nondepressed patient or a nonpatient, Coyne discovered that following a brief conversation, students, not surprisingly, rated depressed patients significantly more negatively than they rated controls. Even more strikingly the students also rated *themselves* as significantly more depressed, anxious and hostile (Coyne, 1976). In a similar study, Hammen and Peters (1977) also found that "depressed" persons were more strongly rejected, especially by persons of the opposite sex. Again, depressed subjects elicited higher ratings of depression in those who conversed with them. Clearly, depression has a dramatic impact on those who come into contact with it, even for brief periods. The negative interactions which are likely to occur as a result of depressive symptoms will no doubt have a greater impact on family members, since they are exposed to them so much more intensively. For couples whose marriages are already troubled, or families with other preexisting problems, this impact may be particularly destructive. There is evidence that if a marriage is distressed, negative communications by one spouse are significantly more likely to be reciprocated by negative communications from the other, and to be related to a decrease in general marital satisfaction (Gottman, 1979; Margolin & Wampol, 1979; Billings & Moos, 1982).

Marital satisfaction, while always important, is particularly relevant for those who are depressed. The quality of the marital relationship has an impact on the likehood of the development of depression and on the course of the illness (Brown & Harris, 1978; Weissman & Paykel, 1974). Several investigators have stressed the value of a confiding relationship (usually with a husband) in protecting women from experiencing depression following negative life events (Brown et al., 1977; Costello, 1982; Roy, 1978). The lack of such a relationship has been noted to increase the likelihood of depression dramatically in a working class population. Four percent of those women with a good relationship became depressed after a negative life event, whereas 42% of those without such a relationship became depressed (Brown et al., 1977). Whether this association is a causal one is unclear. It is possible, for instance, that the absence of such protective relationships in the lives of these women is a *consequence* of low grade chronic depression, or that negative life events for some of these women take on added significance because they occur in the context of already troubled relationships. Nevertheless, these data add cumulative weight to the notion that the quality of existing relationships is relevant for those who are depressed. There is at least beginning evidence that a positive marital relationship predicts the patient's response to treatment.

Even for depressed people whose marriages were previously satisfying, it is likely that their spouses will come to be increasingly frustrated and dissatisfied over time and higher divorce rates will be experienced (Merikangas, 1984). Unfortunately, there has been little attention to the needs and problems of the spouses of depressed individuals (Coyne et al., 1985). In our own small pilot study of patients hospitalized for affective disorders, spouses rated their marriages considerably more negatively than did patients (Anderson et al., in preparation). This finding may reflect the difficulty of living with someone with depressive symptoms. Living with someone who is depressed may be particularly stressful if the partner views the patient's behavior as willful and therefore makes negative attributions about the symptoms over time. Lowered vitality may appear to be laziness; feelings of worthlessness to be self-indulgence; hopelessness and helplessness, unwarranted and excessive; requests for continuous reassurance and comfort may seem unreasonable; and the increasing stridency may seem to be just plain nastiness.

It is only natural that spouses and family members of depressed individuals may become increasingly distressed over time. The fact

that spouses are also likely to be psychiatrically ill, may further complicate the family situation. As many as 60% of patients with affective
disorders appear to be married to a spouse who is also disturbed (Merikangas, 1982). While these statistics may reflect assortive mating,
they may also support an hypothesis about the stress of depressive
interaction. In this regard, the likelihood of the presence of psychiatric
disorders or symptoms in both spouses increases the longer one of
them has been ill and is associated with a significantly less favorable
treatment outcome for the identified patient (Merikangas et al., 1983;
Merikangas et al., 1979; Nelson et al., 1970).

The impact of depressed individuals and distressed marital relationships is not confined to the mental health of the adults in the family,
but is likely to include the children as well. Depressed mothers have
been noted to be less available, less nurturant, to have more problematic relationships with their children than other mothers (Orvaschel, in
press; Weissman, 1972). They have described themselves as having
more friction with their children, less affective involvement and more
communication difficulties (Weissman et al., 1972). They also
seemed to have more resentment and hostility toward their adolescents, required more nurturance *from* them, and were less able to set
limits on their behavior. Perhaps as a result, the children of depressed
women have been described as at increased risk for psychological
problems and even accidents (Brown et al., 1977). The adolescent
children of depressed mothers appear to have more school problems,
more drug abuse, more acting out and more contact with the law
(Weissman & Siegel, 1972). Children of depressed parents have been
found to be three times more likely to receive DSM-III diagnoses than
children of normals (Weissman et al., 1984). While as many as 15%
of children have been noted to be symptomatic if one parent was depressed, those with two parents with psychiatric symptoms experienced twice the incidence of school and psychological problems. Children aged six to seventeen seem to be particularly vulnerable to
parental depression (Weissman et al., 1984). Furthermore, both the
children and the spouses of depressed patients have been reported to
have more visits to their family doctor for physical complaints (Widmer et al., 1980).

TREATMENT: RESEARCH STUDIES

Since depression is often chronic or recurrent, modifying the interactional patterns in these families is likely to be a difficult task. Even
in relatively acute depressions, once negative interactional patterns are

established between spouses they are slow to resolve after depressive symptoms have remitted (Bothwell & Weissman, 1977; Paykel et al., 1969; Weissman & Klerman, 1972). There is some suggestion that relationship problems do improve when symptoms abate, but women in particular tend to report negative marital interactions long after they have recovered from the acute symptoms of depression (Hinchliffe et al., 1975; Hinchliffe et al., 1978) Even children continue to have psychosocial and school problems after depressive symptoms have been successfully treated with medication (Puig-Antich et al., 1986).

These factors support the adoption of a systems orientation in treating depression, focusing on the interpersonal context in which the disorder develops, and the needs of others in the intimate environments of depressed patients. It is particularly striking, therefore, that most of the clinical and research work on depressed patients has had an individual orientation. In fact, only two approaches to the therapy of depressed patients have been shown to be effective and supported by repeated controlled studies, and both are individually oriented.

One approach, cognitive behavioral therapy, widely recognized as an effective treatment approach for depression (Bonine, 1966; Blackburn et al., 1981; Jarvik et al., 1982; Kovacs, 1980; Rush et al., 1980; Rush et al., 1975; Schmickley, 1976; Beck et al., 1961) is based on the assumption that cognition, rather than mood, is central in depression (Zeiss et al., 1979; Beck, 1976). A negative self-image, external events, and the future are thought to prevent a realistic testing of ideas, adaptive problem solving and the judicious use of help and advice. Thus, the core problems in depression are assumed to be idiosyncratic, negative, thought processes which maintain negative self-concepts and negative world views (Beck, 1976).

Cognitive therapy aims to correct maladaptive perceptions and cognitions, and thereby to decrease depressive symptomatology. The course of treatment is generally short-term, usually limited to 20 individual sessions (Beck et al., 1979; Rush et al., 1977; Shaw, 1977). Results of controlled studies include a significant, if temporary, superiority to social skills training, assessment alone, and a no treatment control group (Rush et al., 1977); equal effectiveness to drug treatment (imipramine) on some variables and superior effectiveness on others (Beck et al., 1979); a more powerful effect on self-concept and the reduction of hopelessness than amitriptyline (Shaw, 1977); superior effectiveness to an insight oriented group and a wait list control (Roy, 1978); no major differences with two types of behavior treatment (Beck et al., 1961; Rush & Beck, 1978); superiority alone and in combination with drugs to drugs alone (Bonine, 1966). In the major

NIMH collaborative study comparing cognitive behavioral therapy, interpersonal psychotherapy (IPT), drug therapy (imipramine) and placebo, initial reports indicate that there are no major differences between the effects of psychotherapy and medication, but that medication worked faster (Elkin et al., 1986).

The second method of psychotherapy demonstrated to be effective with depressed patients is Interpersonal Psychotherapy (IPT) developed by Weissman and her colleagues at Yale (Lewinsohn et al., 1980; Weissman, 1979). This approach is based on the assumption that current and future episodes of depression can be alleviated by helping patients to understand their relationships and to develop more effective interpersonal skills. The primary targets of this approach are the symptoms and social adjustment of patients rather than either their thought processes or personalities (Lewinsohn et al., 1980). In this approach, specific techniques were designed to help patients manage loss, interpersonal deficits and role disputes. Despite its interpersonal focus, however, neither the spouse nor other family members are included in the process of treatment. Thus, the therapist is both dependent on the perceptions of the identified patient and unable to intervene directly in negative sequences of interaction between family members.

Nevertheless, controlled trials have demonstrated the superiority of IPT to both no-treatment and to low-contact controls in relieving certain aspects of depression. Additive effects have been found with drug treatments (Weissman, 1979; Weissman et al., 1979). However, there is evidence that even when medication improves mood, marital problems remain (Klerman & Weissman, 1982). While impaired communication and interpersonal friction continue to be a problem for many of these patients after the completion of treatment, this method shows promise in preventing relapse, and in some cases, in improving social functioning (Weissman & Paykel, 1974). However, since women who present with marital disputes are reported to have higher relapse rates, less improvement in both depressive symptoms and social functioning, and a persistent tendency towards continued marital disputes (even when they divorce and form new relationships) (Klerman et al., 1974; Bothwell & Weissman, 1977) it would appear that the effectiveness of IPT in improving relationships is somewhat limited. Studies of the impact of cognitive-behavioral therapy have not tended to measure these factors, but there is no reason to believe that it is any more effective than IPT in improving functioning in this area. Direct attention to relationship issues in depression would seem to be essential. In fact, attempts are being made to develop marital interventions based on each of these treatment approaches, but results of controlled trials are still in the future.

In the family field, currently, only two controlled studies have employed marital therapy with depressed patients, and none has employed family therapy. The earliest and best known controlled study is that of Friedman (1975), involving 196 patients described as having neurotic depressions in a 12 week trial of drug (amitriptyline) or placebo, minimal contact or marital therapy in a 2 × 2 design. Drug therapy was superior to and faster than marital therapy in improving the patient's symptoms. Marital therapy was superior to drug therapy in improving performance of family roles, and in changing perceptions of the spouse's attitudes and behaviors. Global self-report measures of psychosocial functioning revealed the greatest improvement in the combined drug and marital group. This study was also significant in that the investigators reportedly lost few subjects based on the spouse's unwillingness to cooperate, challenging a long-held myth about the vicissitudes of compliance with marital therapy when one spouse is defined as psychiatrically ill. Unfortunately, this study had a number of methodological weaknesses including the fact that the marital intervention used was not described in sufficient detail to allow for replication, and the fact that the study did not control for the sex of the patient. This is particularly unfortunate because there are gender differences in the incidence of depression and different family problems are likely to occur based on the sex of the spouse who happens to become depressed (Hammen & Peters, 1977; Hinchcliffe, 1978). Specifically, marriage and family life will be disrupted differently dependent on which spouse's roles and behaviors are curtailed by the illness, and different behaviors are likely to be tolerated in men and women.

More recently, behaviorally oriented marital therapy, involving either communication problem solving training and/or behavior exchange techniques, have been examined in a variety of studies, beginning now to include those suffering from depression. The problem solving approach to behavioral marital therapy seems particularly useful in maintaining change over time (Jacobson, 1982). After spending many years developing and refining the techniques of a behavioral marital therapy model with more mildly distressed couples, Jacobson applied these methods of intervention to the marriages of six couples in which one partner was a psychiatric patient (Jacobson, 1982; Jacobson et al., 1980). Although the numbers were small and the patients were not necessarily depressed (or even meeting criteria for any particular psychiatric disorder), all six couples were reported as improved by the end of treatment and five had maintained these gains at follow-up (Jacobson et al., 1980). This same investigator is currently conducting a more extensive study of behavioral marital therapy with women who meet criteria for major depression, comparing behavioral marital therapy (BMT), cognitive-behavioral therapy for the patient alone (CBT), both treatments concurrently, and a minimal contact control (Jacobson, 1982).

TREATMENT: CLINICAL DESCRIPTIONS

Coyne (1984, 1986) has proposed a method of strategic marital therapy for depression. Based on the assumption that depression arises from the use of inappropriate coping strategies in dealing with everyday problems or life transitions by depressed individuals and their significant others, this method of treatment attempts to interrupt current ineffective interactional sequences in the marriage. Interventions are focused in three areas: the distress of the depressed person, the spouse's response, and the marital relationship. Strategic maneuvers directed at the patient include respecting the individual's right to remain depressed, emphasizing the drawbacks of improved functioning, and the function of the patient's depression in protecting a vulnerable spouse. Maneuvers with the spouse include modulating the tendencies toward over and under involvement in the relationship, prescribed disagreements, and relabels. While this method has theoretical and clinical appeal, it has not yet been supported by research using controlled clinical trials.

Elsewhere (Anderson et al., 1986), I have presented the results of a beginning attempt to apply a psychoeducational intervention first developed for use with chronic schizophrenia patients and their families (the content of which was based in part upon Coyne's observations of problematic interactional sequences) with families of patients with affective disorders. Forty inpatients with affective disorders, primarily with a diagnosis of depression were randomly assigned to a process oriented multiple family group, or a psychoeducational group emphasizing the provision of information about the patients' illness and methods of coping with it effectively. Measures were taken pre- and post-group sessions, but no attempt was made to do follow-up measures or control other treatments. Very few changes in knowledge or attitude were found following the sessions and no attempt was made to actually measure changes in coping. Those attending the psychoeducational sessions, however, reported significantly more satisfaction with the experience. Minimally psychoeducational measures might thus encourage family support of the patients treatment and thus increase treatment complicance in patients. A more extensive and sustained clinical research program would be necessary to determine whether these interventions could possibly influence family relationships and/or the course of the disorder.

DISCUSSION AND SUMMARY

Depression is correlated with significant family dysfunction, including marital problems, disturbed communication and decreased sexual and marital satisfaction. Both children and spouses of depressed individuals seem to become symptomatic over time. Whether this is due to the tendency of depressed individuals to choose one another as partners, and/or presenting genetic/biological variables as opposed to the impact of symptoms, stress and ineffective or exhausted methods of coping is unclear. Reports also are mixed as to whether or not marital/family problems improve as symptoms remit, but indications are that improved family relationships are more likely for male patients than female ones. In any case, families with good functioning before the onset of depression appear to have better long-term outcomes than those with preexisting problems. Family factors, in other words, do seem to have an influence on the course of the disorder. Findings from epidemiological studies are conflicting, but indicate that early loss and current support play a role in the onset or incidence of the disorder.

While family and marital problems no doubt have a role in the onset, course and outcome of the disorder, specific conclusions must be regarded as tentative due to universal methodological problems with existing studies. Criteria for defining depression, small samples, self-report methodology, lack of attention to the timing of measures (during or between episodes), absence of control groups, and reliance on retrospective reports, all influence the quality of ratings of the characteristics of depressed subjects and their families. Furthermore, few attempts have been made to design and investigate family/marital intervention despite the fact that families influence and are seriously influenced by the disorder. Methods of some promise include behavioral marital therapy, strategic marital therapy, a couples version of interpersonal psychotherapy, and psychoeducational interventions. Studies of the possible effectiveness of these treatments are needed if we are to design and implement programs to help the large numbers of individuals and families whose lives are disrupted by depression.

REFERENCES

Akiskal, H. S., Bitar, A. H., Puzantian, V. R., Rosenthal, T. L., Walker, P. W. The nosological status of neurotic depression: A prospective 3 to 4 year follow-up examination in light of the primary-secondary and unipolar-bipolar dichotomies. *Archives of General Psychiatry*, 35, 6, 1978, 756-766.

Anderson, C., Hogarty, G. & Reiss, D. Family treatment of adult schizophrenic patients: A psychoeducational approach. *Schizophrenia Bulletin*, 6, 3, 1980, 490-505.

Anderson, C. M., Griffin, S., Rossi, A., Pagonis, I., Holder, D. & Treiber, R. A comparative study of the impact of education vs. process groups for families of patients with affective disorders. *Family Process*, 1986.

Andreason, N. C. & Winokur, G. Secondary depression: Familial, clinical and research perspectives. *American Journal of Psychiatry*, 136, 1979, 62-66.

Beck, A. T. *Cognitive therapy and emotional disorders*. New York: International Universities Press, 1976.

Beck, A. T., Rush, A. J., Shaw, B. F. et al. *Cognitive therapy of depression*. New York: Guilford Press, 1979.

Beck, A. T., Ward, C. H., Mendelson, J. et al. An inventory for measuring depression. *Archives of General Psychiatry*, 4, 1961, 561-571.

Billings, A. G. & Moos, R. H. Psychosocial theory and research in depression: An integrative framework and review. *Clinical Psychology Review*, 1, 1982, 213-238.

Blackburn, I., Bishop, S., Glen, A., Whalley, L. & Christie, J. The efficacy of cognitive therapy in depression: A treatment trial using cognitive therapy and pharmacotherapy, each alone and in combination. *British Journal of Psychiatry*, 139, 1981, 181-189.

Blatt, S. J., Wein, S. J., Chevron, E. & Quinlan, D. M. Parental representations and depression in normal young adults. *Journal of Abnormal Psychology*, 88, 4, 1976, 388-397.

Bonine, W. Depression as a practice: Dynamics and psychotherapeutic considerations. *Comprehensive Psychiatry*, 1, 1960, 194-201.

Bonine, W. The psychodynamics of neurotic depression. In S. Arieti (Ed.), *American handbook of psychiatry, vol. 3*. New York: Basic Books, 1966.

Bothwell, S. & Weissman, M. Social impairments four years after an acute depressive episode. *American Journal of Orthopsychiatry*, 47, 2, 1977, 231-237.

Briscoe, C. W. & Smith, J. B. Depression & marital turmoil. *Archives of General Psychiatry*, 29, 1973, 811-817.

Bromet, E. J. & Cornley, P. J. Correlates of depression in mothers of young children. *Journal of the American Academy of Child Psychiatry*, 23, 3, 1984, 335-342.

Brown, G. W. & Harris, T. O. *Social origins of depression: A study of psychiatric disorder in women*. New York: Free Press, 1978.

Brown, G. W., Harris, T. & Copland, J. R. Depression and loss. *British Journal of Psychiatry*, 130, 1977, 1-18.

Cammer, L. Family feedback in depressive illnesses. *Psychosomatics*, 12, 1971, 127-132.

Collins, J., Kreitman, N., Nelson, B. & Troop, J. Neurosis and marital interaction: III. Family roles & functions. *British Journal of Psychiatry*, 119, 1971, 233-242.

Costello, C. G. Social factors associated with depression: A retrospective community study. *Psychological Medicine*, 12, 1982, 329-339.

Coyne, J. C. Depression & the response of others. *Journal of Abnormal Psychology*, 1976, 85, 186-193.

Coyne, J. C. Strategic marital therapy for depression. In N. S. Jacobson & A. S. Gurman (Eds.) *Clinical handbook of marital therapy*. New York: Guilford Press, 1986, 495-511.

Coyne, J. C. Strategic therapy with married depressed persons: Initial agenda, themes and interventions. *Journal of Marital and Family Therapy*, 10, 1984, 53-62.

Coyne, J. C., Kahn, J. & Gotlib, I. Depression. In T. Jacob (Ed.), *Family interaction and psychopathology*. New York: Pergamon Press, 1985.

Eidelson, R. J. & Epstein, N. Cognition & relationship maladjustment: Development of a measure of dysfunctional relationship beliefs. *Journal of Consulting & Clinical Psychology*, 50, 5, 1982, 715-720.

Elkin, I., Shea, T., Watkins, J., Imber, S., Sotsky, S., Collins, J., Glass, D., Pilkonis, P., Leber, W., Ferster, S., Docherty, J., Parloff, M. NIMH Collaborative research program: General effectiveness of treatment. Paper presented to the Society for Psychotherapy Research, June, 1986.

Falloon, I. R., Boyd, J. L., McGill, C. W., Razani, J., Moss, H. B. &, Gilderman, A. M. Family management in the prevention of exacerbations of schizophrenia. *New England Journal of Medicine*, 306, June, 1982, 1437-1440.

Friedman, A. S. Interaction of drug therapy with marital therapy in depressive patients. *Archives of General Psychiatry*, 32, May, 1975, 619-637.

Gallagher, W. The dark affection of mind and body. *Discover*, May, 1986, 66-76.

Goering, P. N., Lancee, W. J. & Freeman, S. J. J. Expressed emotions and recovery from depression. Paper presented at the annual meeting of the American Psychiatric Association. Los Angeles, May, 1984.

Goldstein, M. & Kopeikin, H. Short and long term effects of combining drug and family therapy. In M. J. Goldstein (Ed.), *New developments in interventions with families of schizophrenics*, San Francisco, Jossey-Bass, 1981.

Golin, S., Sweeney, P. & Shaeffer, D. The causality of causal attributions in depression: A cross-logged panel correlational analysis. *Journal of Abnormal Psychology*, 90, 1, 1981, 14-22.

Gottman, J. M. *Marital interaction: Experimental investigations*. New York: Academic Press, 1979.

Hammen, C. L. & Peters, S. D. Differential response to male and female depressive reactions. *Journal of Consulting and Clinical Psychology*, 45, 1977, 994-1001.

Hammen, C. L. & Peters, S. D. Interpersonal consequences of depression. Responses to men and women enacting a depressed role. *Journal of Abnormal Psychology*, 87, 322-332.

Hinchcliffe, M., Hooper, D., Roberts, F. J. & Pamela, W. V. A study of the interaction between depressed patients & their spouses. *British Journal of Psychiatry*, 126, 1975, 164-172.

Hinchcliffe, M. K., Hooper, D. & Roberts, F. J. *The melancholy marriage: Depression in marriage & psychosocial approaches to therapy*. New York: Wiley, 1978.

Hoover, C. F. & Fitzgerald, R. G. Dominance in the marriages of affective patients. *Journal of Nervous & Mental Disease*, 169, 10, 1981, 624-628.

Hops, H., Beglan, A., Sherman, L., Arthur, J. & Friedman, L.S. Direct observation study of family processes in maternal depression. Paper presented at the annual convention of the American Psychological Association, Anaheim, California, 1983.

Jacobson, N. S. Behavioral marital therapy and treatment of depression. Grant submitted to NIMH, 1982.

Jacobson, N. S., Waldron, H. & Moore, D. Toward a behavioral profile of marital distress. *Journal of Consulting and Clinical Psychology*, 48, 1980, 696-703.

Jarvik, L. F., Mintz, J., Stever, J. & Gerner, R. Treating geriatric depression: A 26 week interim analysis. *Journal of the American Geriatrics Society*, 1982, 713-717.

Keitner, G., Baldwin, L., Epstein, N. & Bishop, D. Family functioning in patients with affective disorder. A review. *International Journal of Family Psychiatry*. In press.

Klerman, G. L., DiMascio, A., Weissman, M. M., Prusoff, B. & Paykal, E. S. Treatment of depression by drugs and psychotherapy. *American Journal of Psychiatry*, 131, 1974, 186-191.

Klerman, G. L. & Weissman, M. M. Interpersonal psychology and theory . . . Research. In A. J. Rush (Ed.), *Short term psychotherapy for depression: Behavioral, interpersonal, cognitive and psychodynamic approaches*. New York: Guilford Press, 1982.

Kovacs, M. The efficacy of cognitive and behavior therapies for depression. *The American Journal of Psychiatry*, 137, 1980, 1495-1501.

Leff, J. & Vaughn, C. The role of maintenance therapy and relatives' expressed emotion in relapse of schizophrenia: A two year follow-up. *British Journal of Psychiatry*, 139, 1981, 102-104.

Lewine, R., Watt, N., Prentky, R. & Fryer, J. Childhood behavior in schizophrenia, personality disorder, depression & neurosis. *British Journal of Psychiatry*, 133, 1978, 347-357.

Lewinsohn, P. M., Mischel, W., Chaplin, W. & Barton, R. Social competence and depression: The role of illusory self-perceptions. *Journal of Abnormal Psychology*, 89, 1980, 203-212.

McCranie, E. J. Depression, anxiety and hostility. *Psychiatric Quarterly*, 45, 1971, 117-133.

McLean, P. D. & Hakistan, A. R. Clinical depression: Comparative efficacy of outpatient treatments. *Journal of Consulting and Clinical Psychology*, 47, 1979, 818-836.

Margolin, G. & Wampol, J. B. Sequential analysis of conflict and accord in distressed and nondistressed marital partners. *Journal of Consulting and Clinical Psychology*, 47, 1979, 368-376.

Merikangas, K. Divorce and assortive mating among depressed patients. *American Journal of Psychiatry*, 141, 1, 1984, 74-76.

Merikangas, K. R. Assortative mating for psychiatric disorders & psychological traits. *Archives of General Psychiatry*, 39, 1982, 1173-1180.

Merikangas, K. R., Bromet, E. J. & Spiker, D. G. The relationship of assortive mating to social adjustment and course of illness in primary affective disorder. *Archives of General Psychiatry*, 40, 1983, 795-800.

Merikangas, K. R., Prusoff, B., Kupfer, D. & Frank, E. Marital adjustment in major depression. *Journal of Affective Disorder*, 9, 5-11, 1985.

Merikangas, K. R., Ranelli, C. J. & Kupfer, D. J. Marital interaction in hospitalized depressed patients. *Journal of Nervous & Mental Disease*, 167, 11, 1979, 689-695.

Nelson, B., Collins, J., Kreitman, N. & Troop, J. Neurosis and marital interaction II: Trust sharing and social activity. *British Journal of Psychiatry*, 117, 1970, 47-58.

Orvaschel, H. Maternal depression & child dysfunction: Children at risk. In B. Lahey and A. Kazdin (Eds.), *Advances in Clinical Child Psychology, Vol. 6*. New York: Academia Press. In press.

Parker, G. Parental characteristics in relation to depressive disorders. *British Journal of Psychiatry*, 134, 1979, 138-147.

Paykel, E. S., Myers, J. K., Dienelt, M. N., Klerman, G. L., Lindenthal, J. J. & Pepper, M. P. Life events and depression: A controlled study. *Archives of General Psychiatry*, 21, 1969, 753-760.

Perris, C. Personality patterns in patients with affective disorders. *American Journal of Psychiatry*, 221, 1971, 43-51.

Puig-Antich, J., Lukens, E., Davies, M., Goetz, D. & Todak, G. Psychosocial functioning in prepubertal major depressive disorders. II. Interpersonal relationships after sustained recovery from affective episode. *Archives of General Psychiatry*, 42, 1985, 511-517.

Rosenthal, T. L., Hagop, S. A., Scott-Strauss, A., Rosenthal, R. H. & Bavia, M. Familial & developmental factors in characteriological depressions. *Journal of Affective Disorders*, 3, 1981, 183-192.

Rounsaville, B. J., Prusoff, B. A. & Weissman, M. M. The course of marital disputes in depressed women: a 48 month follow up study. *Comprehensive Psychiatry*, 21, 2, 1980, 111-118.

Roy, A. The role of past loss in depression. *Archives of General Psychiatry*, 38, 1981, 301-302.

Roy, A. Vulnerability factors & depression in women. *British Journal of Psychiatry*, 133, 1978, 106-10.

Rush, A. J. & Beck, A. T. Adults with affective disorders. In M. Hersen & A. Bellack (Eds.), *Behavior Therapy in the Psychiatric Setting*. Baltimore: Williams & Wilkins Co., 1978.

Rush, A. J., Beck, A. T., Kovacs, M. & Hollon, S. Comparative efficacy of cognitive therapy and imipramine in the treatment of depressed outpatients. *Cognitive Therapy and Research*, 1, 1977, 17-37.

Rush, A. J., Khatami, M. & Beck, A. T. Cognitive and behavior therapy in chronic depression. *Behavior Therapy*, 6, 1975, 398-404.

Rush, A. J., Shaw, B. & Khatami, M. Cognitive therapy of depression: Utilizing the couples system. *Cognitive Therapy & Research*, 4, 1, 1980, 103-113.

Schmickley, V. G. The effects of cognitive-behavior modification upon depressed outpatients. Doctoral dissertation, Michigan State University, 1976.

Seligman, M., Abramson, L., Semmel, A. & van Baeyer, C. Depressive attributional style. *Journal of Abnormal Psychology*, 88, 3, 1979, 242-247.

Shaw, B. A comparison of cognitive therapy and behavior therapy in the treatment of depression. *Journal of Consulting and Clinical Psychology*, 45, 1977, 543-551.

Spitzer, R. L., Endicott, J. & Robins, E. Research and diagnostic criteria: Rationale and reliability. *Archives of General Psychiatry*, 35, 1978, 773-778.

Vaughn, C. E. & Leff, J. P. Influence of family & social factors on the course of psychiatric illness. *British Journal of Psychiatry*, 129, 1976, 125-127.

Weissman, M. The depressed woman: Recent research. *Social Work*, Sept. 1972, 19-25.

Weissman, M. M. The psychological treatment of depression: Evidence for the efficacy of psychotherapy alone, in comparison with and in combination with pharmacotherapy. *Archives of General Psychiatry*, 36, 1979, 1261-1269.

Weissman, M. M. & Akiskal, H. S. The role of psychotherapy in chronic depression: A proposal. *Comprehensive Psychiatry*, 25, 1, 1984, 23-31.

Weissman, M. M. & Klerman, G. L. Sex differences and the epidemiology of depression. *Archives of General Psychiatry*, 34, 1972, 98-111.

Weissman, M. M. & Paykel, E. S. *The depressed woman: A study of social relationships*. Chicago: University of Chicago Press, 1974.

Weissman, M. M. Prusoff, B. A., DiMascio, A., Neu, C. & Goklaney, M. The efficacy of drugs and psychotherapy in the treatment of acute depressive episodes. *American Journal of Psychiatry*, 136, 1979, 555-558.

Widmer, R. B., Codoret, R. J. & North, C. S. Depression in family practice: Some effects on spouses and children. *The Journal of Family Practice*, 1980, 10, 1, 45-51.

Zeiss, A. M., Lewinsohn, P. M. & Munoz, R. F. Nonspecific improvement effects in depression using interpersonal skills training, pleasant activity schedules, or cognitive training. *Journal of Consulting and Clinical Psychology*, 47, 1979, 427-439.

Borderline Disorders:
Family Assessment and Treatment

Craig A. Everett
Sandra S. Volgy

Most family therapists who began practicing a decade or more ago found, as we did, that there were few guidelines and even fewer models available in the literature which linked assessment and treatment into a coherent clinical strategy. However, most of us knew that as we were trying to understand what a "systemic paradigm" meant in clinical practice and as we shifted our "epistemological" position away from our early individually-oriented training, we were discovering pieces of the larger puzzle of human behavior that the prevailing literature had never conceptualized.

In the area of severe and chronic emotional disorders, there had been a few "landmark" studies identifying the schizophrenogenic family and positing the double-bind theory. However, other areas of traditional psychiatric classification had been virtually ignored by family therapists. In 1978, along with our other colleagues, we were treating diagnosed borderline individuals in the context of their families. As we shared our observations, we began to recognize similar structural and interactive patterns within these family systems. As we collected and compared more clinical data, it became apparent that by looking beyond the traditional presenting symptoms of a borderline individual, it was possible to identify and even predict patterns intrinsic to the family system in which they lived.

Craig A. Everett, PhD, is Associate Professor and Director of Family Therapy Training in the Interdivisional Program in Marriage and Family, Florida State University, Tallahassee, FL 32306. He is in private practice with the Southeast Family Institute. Sandra S. Volgy, PhD, is Clinical Psychologist, Family Therapist and Mediator in private practice with the Southeast Family Institute, 1640 Metropolitan Circle, Tallahassee, FL 32308. She is also Adjunct Clinical Supervisor with the Interdivisional Program at Florida State University.

This paper highlights material from the forthcoming work, *The Borderline Family: Systemic Assessment and Treatment*, C. Everett, S. Halperin, S. Volgy, and Anne Wissler. New York: Grune & Stratton, in press.

As we defined and conceptualized these dynamics further, we also began to recognize that interactive patterns identical to those that we had found appeared in other clinical families where there was no diagnosed or identifiable borderline individual. These findings led us into a project that has spanned over eight years and the collection of clinical data on over 200 borderline families from a variety of treatment settings. This paper will highlight the major assessment and treatment issues which are discussed and illustrated in the report of this study: Everett, Halperin, Volgy, and Wissler, in press.

THE PSYCHIATRIC DEFINITION

Considerable debate has occurred in the psychiatric literature over the past two decades regarding issues of classification and differential diagnosis for the borderline condition. Discussions have ranged from identifying it as a clinical syndrome, to a characterological pattern, to a form of personality organization, to the more recently preferred "condition." Gunderson and Singer (1975) traced the concept's development from Bleuler's "latent schizophrenia" (1911) to Zilborg's "ambulatory schizophrenia" (1941) to Deutsch's "as if personality" (1942). These evolved into the preferred classification of "pseudoneurotic schizophrenia" until the more recent shift to borderline.

Similarly, clinical efforts to identify specific assessment features have varied widely in the psychiatric literature. An analysis by Perry and Klerman (1978) of four such published efforts identified 104 different assessment criteria. A study of 160 practicing psychiatrists reported the diagnostic variation of "borderline psychotic" among clients up to 12 years of age and "borderline personality" for clients between 12 and 18 years of age (Bradley, 1981).

Perhaps the most widely cited classification of borderline assessment features was developed by Gunderson and Singer (1975). They identified six characteristics:

1. minipsychotic episodes or brief lapses of reality testing;
2. the presence of intense affect such as anger, hostility, or emptiness;
3. a certain social adaptiveness;
4. a history of impulsive behavior;
5. loose thinking in unstructured situations;
6. relationships that vacillate between transient superficiality and intense dependency.

The decision to include the borderline designation in the third edition of the *Diagnostic and Statistical Manual of Mental Disorders* (APA, 1980) served both to legitimize this condition as an acceptable psychiatric diagnosis and to bring some definition regarding its assessment features. The *DSM III* has identified eight criteria which can be summarized as follows: impulsivity or unpredictability, unstable and intense interpersonal relationships, inappropriate and intense anger, uncertainty regarding issues of identity and self-image, affective instability, intolerance of being alone, physically self-damaging acts, chronic feelings of emptiness or boredom.

The etiological understanding of the borderline condition in psychiatric literature evolves from object relations theory (see Jacobson, 1964; Guntrip, 1969, Blanck & Blanck, 1974; Kernberg, 1976; and Mahler, 1971, 1975). Most of the literature follows Mahler's (1971, 1975) developmental framework (i.e., autism, symbiosis, separation-individuation, object constancy) which places the timing of the dysfunctional elements in the rapprochement subphase of the separation-individuation stage. This is a period between 16 and 25 months where the infant is struggling to establish preliminary boundaries from the mother. The infant's typical behavior of shadowing and darting away from the adult characterizes an internal struggle between a wish for reunion and a fear of engulfment.

When the milieu offered by the mother is experienced as erratic, ranging from clinging to withdrawal, the normal developmental crisis is exacerbated. This increases aggression in the infant which is experienced by the mother as coercion. Kernberg (1975) observed that this rage toward the mother must be internalized as an image of a bad child being abandoned by an angry mother in order for the child to cling to an external fantasy of the mother as good and rewarding. These patterns are the roots of the typical splitting and projective dynamics of the borderline adult.

With the failure to achieve object constancy, the infant continues to perceive his/her world as unpredictable and frightening: "He sees his heroes develop feet of clay as he repeatedly idealizes them and is inevitably disappointed; tiny frustrations assume the dimensions of catastrophes, with ensuing eruption of disproportionately strong affects, often rage" (Carter & Rinsley, 1977, p. 317).

These factors lead to the development of the primary constellation of defenses in the borderline condition: splitting and projective identification. The primitive mechanism of splitting allows the borderline individual to manage the intolerable ambivalence in relationships by separating the representation of the objects into all "good" and all "bad." This preambivalent state protects the individual's weak ego structure from inherent frustrations and contradictions in both past and present relationships. The resultant lack of integrated object representations characterizes the borderline individual's limited capacity for understanding and empathy in a relationship (Masterson & Rinsley, 1975), and explains the abrupt shifts between "good" and "bad" perceptions which are a part of the individual's mood instability (Kernberg, 1975).

Projective identification, which occurs along a broad range of interaction, involves the projection of unacceptable aspects of the self onto another person in a close relationship and the resultant identification with, or reaction to, those attributes accepted by the other individual. This mechanism is utilized by the borderline individual to control the danger perceived in close relationships. The borderline individual will try to evoke behavior in the other person that confirms the projection while at the same time the other accepts these projected attributes as part of himself/herself. The resultant identification after the projection occurs because of the weak ego boundaries of the borderline individual. Kernberg (1975) has suggested that the borderline individual continues to experience these projected parts and thus fears and must control the other individual who has accepted them.

FAMILIAL PATTERNS IN CLINICAL RESEARCH: A TRANSGENERATIONAL MODEL

There is no literature available which offers an integrative statement of family dynamics pertaining either to the development of the borderline condition or resultant patterns within the nuclear family. However, from the limited clinical data reported, it is possible to organize a preliminary model identifying intergenerational patterns of development.

There are a few studies which have analyzed comparative familial data of borderline individuals with that of other diagnostic groupings. Most of these studies concur that the borderline condition evolves in a milieu of family turmoil and disorganization. Gunderson et al., (1980) compared family assessment data among inpatient young adults (15 to 24 years of age) diagnosed respectively as borderline, paranoid schizophrenic, and neurotic. They reported that the families of the borderline individuals, in contrast to the neurotic group, displayed poorer enforcement of rules and a higher incidence of maternal psychosis and ineffectiveness. In contrast to the schizophrenic group, the borderline families evidenced greater maternal depression and psychosis. Overall, the parents of the borderline young adults were less functional than the comparison groups and their marriages were characterized by an absence of overt conflict and a quality of attachment that seemed to exclude the children.

In a similar analysis, Walsh (1977) compared family data on borderline and schizophrenic inpatients. She reported that the borderline group displayed a lower frequency of intact families of origin and that one-half of this group displayed serious parental illness (mental and physical) requiring extended or multiple hospitalizations. Grinker and Werble (1968) reported that borderline individuals tended to characterize their families of origin as "not a mutually protective unit," and the family functioning was characterized by discord, confusion and conflict.

These studies, while limited, reflect an important attempt to characterize familial patterns in borderline development. Other clinical reports provide numerous observations of intergenerational features and patterns. Based on an extensive review of the available clinical literature (reported elsewhere, Everett, Halperin, Volgy, & Wissler, in press) and the data collected from this project, we will present here a summary model of familial development.

It is our observation, overall, that borderline development occurs in a multigenerational enmeshing and centripetal system. This is supported by numerous references to ineffective separation and individuation patterns throughout the system. Despite erratic patterns in parent-child attachment, members of these systems are bound tightly by vertical loyalties to their respective families of origin.

This is true in the parents of the borderline whose relationship is characterized by a needy, yet dominating female who selects a passive and often distant male. This complementarity produces a pseudo-mutual relationship which appears tension-free and dependent but which lacks integration and attachment with a blurring of marital and parental boundaries. The wife appears to have had the more fragmented emotional development with more observable dysfunctions ranging from emotional preoccupation and unavailability to psychosis and suicide.

The chronic or periodic incapacitation typical of the mother and unavailability of the father set the stage for the triangulation of a child into an intensive parentified role. No pattern of ordinal position has been identified in the selection of the parentified child. This child is destined to become what we have termed the *borderline carrier* because, as will be explained, this individual as an adult may not always display diagnosable borderline symptoms. The parentified child now becomes caught in a confusing and erratic emotional web where both independent activities and dependent needs are alternately denied and solicited by the parents' own unavailability and neediness. This allows the parental marriage to remain at one level "conflict-free."

However, the intensity of the parentified child's role creates a crisis as the need for individuation occurs in late adolescence. The system's need for the role of this child has been reciprocally reinforced and early efforts to individuate and leave home are typically aborted though often associated with suicidal gestures and symptom formation. We should note here that in the great majority of our clinical population the borderline carrier has been identified as the female. It appears easier for female borderline carriers to achieve some separation from family of origin than for males. In the Walsh (1977) and Grinker and Werble (1968) studies we cited previously, all of the males in their samples, while a small number, had never married. (See Everett, Halperin, Volgy and Wissler, in press for a further discussion.)

The highly enmeshing qualities of this system tend to propel the borderline carrier out of the family and into an emotionally premature relationship and marriage, frequently without prior courtship experiences. The complementarity of the mate selection frequently replicates that in the family of origin in the selection of a passive, dependent and ineffective spouse. This spouse either remains closely tied to his/her own family of origin or has "cut-off" those loyalties and becomes an isolated, "loner" figure. The borderline carrier, now typically as wife and potential mother, carries the intensity of her parentified role into the relationships of this new system, often with a resolve to "do better" as a mother than she experienced with her own parents. While this role provides her with the mechanism for continued emotional control, it also carries the internal vulnerability of failure from her family of origin. It is perhaps this vulnerability that intensifies her continuing loyalty and enmeshment with her own parents and family of origin.

DEFINING THE BORDERLINE FAMILY

We indicated that in the early years of this study our attention was directed at diagnoseable borderline individuals within the context of their family systems. After we had identified recognizable and predictable structures in these systems, we began to recognize both with our clients and those of our clinical students, family cases which displayed the same phenomena but where there was no identifiable borderline parent. At first we thought we were just missing a diagnosis. But after careful assessment and consultation it became apparent that these patterns appeared independent of a diagnosed borderline individual. Thus we began to define this as a preliminary systemic typology of family behavior.

Overall, the borderline family can be characterized as the product of intergenerational enmeshment across at least three generations. In the borderline system the differentiation of subsystems and their internal boundaries are diffuse. The parents display continuing high loyalties to their respective families of origin with the resultant lack of personal individuation and separation. Rigid triangulation occurs where typically two children are pulled out of their sibling subsystem and into intense roles required to balance the rest of the system. The emotional core of the system is a collusively held myth that loss and separation are too painful for the system to tolerate and the expression of anger is dangerous and threatening to the survival of the system and its members.

The most striking feature of the borderline family is that the mechanisms of splitting and projective identification are not displayed simply by an individual but pervade the parent-child subsystem. Splitting occurs when positive and negative feelings and thoughts are separated and experienced by family members in isolation of one another. This splitting distorts the family's perception of reality in such a way as to cause them to experience both internal or external events or issues as either "right" or "wrong," "black" or "white."

Such rigidly split perceptions occur without regard to the complexity of situations, roles or relationships. Studies of borderline adolescents identified a similar pattern where within the family system positive attributes of "goodness" and negative attributes of "badness" were separated and reinvested such that "Each family member appears relatively preambivalent and single-minded in relation to the troubled adolescent" (Shapiro et al., 1977, p. 79; Zinner & Shapiro, 1975). This splitting appears to protect the system from potential feelings of loss and disappointment as well as from the negative affects of anger and hostility.

The projective identification process within a system operates in concert with that of splitting to form rigid role assignments and expectations among specific family members. In the borderline system, the threat of conflict or aggression in the marriage, which would also threaten the survival of the system, is projected onto a child who "owns" the projection and behaves more aggressively while returning the spousal subsystem to a calmer level.

In assessing a clinical family, most family therapists would identify a central triangle, typically between parents and a child, which serves to balance the entire system. The role of the triangulated child is often defined by either parentification or scapegoating. It is rare, except in large families of four or more siblings, to locate at a specific point in time more than one central triangle, though other secondary triangles may exist across generations (see Nichols and Everett, 1986).

We have identified in the borderline family predictable patterns of two central triangles and have termed these coexisting triangles. It appears that the unique level of emotional intensity in the borderline family requires multiple central triangles to balance and stabilize the system. They typically take the form of split and projected images of a triangulated "good" child and "bad" child. It appears that the tenuousness of the parental bonding and the continual threat of destructive anger requires two children to perform these specified roles in order to dissipate these threats and to ensure the survival of the system.

Early in our study we had assumed that the triangulated "good" child was simply playing a parentified role. However, as we studied further clinical data, we found this role to be much more complex and redefined it as the *omnipotent/pseudo-parentified child*. This child is perceived as doing no wrong. He/she follows no rules and acts without consequences. While this child has access and power within the spousal subsystem he/she does not perform a truly nurturing or caretaking role as would be expected in a parentified child. While this role of the "good" child existed within every borderline system, though some had left home and continued to play this role, the actual nurturing/caretaking role was controlled by the borderline carrier, typically the mother.

In addition, again unlike the typical parentified child, this omnipotent/pseudo-parentified child does act out, often covertly and manipulatively, but such behavior is never punished. In one case this "good" child was a married, 23-year-old daughter who had been through three abortions before she was 17. She continued to be idealized by the family with a large formal wedding at 19. She lived four blocks away from her parents and dropped by every weekday morning at 7:00 a.m. before work to have coffee with her mother.

The contrasting triangulation of the "bad" child in the borderline system represents a special type of scapegoat. The child accepts the projected anger and conflict as does a typical scapegoat, but instead of simply acting this out in delinquent activities away from the family, this child explicitly turns the anger back onto the family in a *persecuting* and often terrorizing manner. At one level this serves to dissipate the parental stress and reinforce the split-off nature of the anger. At another it keeps the child closely enmeshed with the system, avoids the threat of separation, and yet contains the anger just outside of the spousal subsystem. In one dramatic case, a persecuting child so terrorized the mother and his "omnipotent" brother when the father was out of town on business that they would lock themselves in a bedroom for hours to avoid his wrath. This pattern had repeated itself consistently over a three-year period prior to the family seeking therapy.

As we have noted, the borderline carrier may never be identified as the presenting problem for therapy. In many cases it is the dramatic behavior of the "persecuting" child that is identified for treatment. We have hypothesized that the greater the level of persecutory behavior by this "bad" child, the more intense will be the level of deflected spousal hostility. Similarly, the greater the level of idealization of the "omnipotent" child, the greater will be the emotional distance between the spouses.

These respective omnipotent and persecuting roles in the borderline system were supported by all members of the family and collusively adopted into the mythology of the system. Once established, these roles for the children appear to become rigid and enduring throughout childhood and even after the children have left home and married. In very few cases did these roles rotate among other siblings. If a family had only one child or a second had been removed, it was the role of the "bad" child which typically shifted to the father. In families with more than two children, these excess siblings would leave the system prematurely often as if they were expelled by the intense exclusivity of the two-triangle system.

In general, we have been able to categorize these borderline systems according to the relative degrees of structural flexibility. Low structural flexibility in a system is evident where the projected roles of the children are rigid and set, where the parents are intensely tied to their own families of origin, and where the external boundaries that define the nuclear or intergenerational system are rigidly closed and isolate the family from external input. High structural flexibility is evident where the system adapts more readily to parental movement between nuclear and family of origin systems. This system displays less intensity both in family of origin loyalties and in the enactment of the projected roles of the children. They evidence more permeable external boundaries and greater social contact outside of the family. These relative categories are useful in the development of specific treatment strategies.

DEVELOPING FAMILY THERAPY STRATEGIES

It is, of course, our position that family therapy is the treatment of choice in working with borderline families whether or not the system presents with an identified borderline parent or an acting-out persecuting child. We have discussed elsewhere the continuing difficulties in conducting individual psychotherapy with the borderline condition (Everett, Halperin, Volgy, & Wissler, in press). Such issues are reflected throughout the psychiatric literature.

Based on the experiences of this study, we believe the following clinical goals are appropriate for family therapy with the borderline system:

1. To increase the family's interactive and perceptive abilities for accepting one another within the system and for recognizing that aspects of the external world contain both "good" and "bad" features. This involves the clinical task of decreasing the systemic splitting process.
2. To increase the abilities of all family members to "own" or accept potentially negative aspects of themselves and thus to be able to move toward interacting as "whole" persons with one another. This involves the clinical task of "working through" the interpersonal distortions and reducing the systemic projective identification process.
3. To move the interactional patterns and experiences within the system to a more openly affiliative level. This involves the clinical task of reducing the oppositional and stereotypical role behavior of all of the members, particularly that of the persecuting and pseudo-parentified children.
4. To "reset" external boundaries for both the nuclear and intergenerational systems. This involves the clinical task of "closing" the external boundaries around the nuclear system which will have the effect of reducing the vertical loyalties for both parents.
5. To "reset" the internal nuclear boundaries for the spousal, parent-child, and siblings subsystems. This involves the clinical task of "closing" the internal boundaries between the spousal and the sibling subsystems to limit the reciprocal intrusiveness of the children and the parents with one another. This will result in a clearer alliance between the two parents.

To operationalize these goals in family therapy, clear strategies must be developed which reflect the patterns and dynamics outlined in the assessment data. The discussion here will focus on outpatient family therapy. The implementation of family therapy with borderline families in an inpatient setting has been discussed elsewhere (Everett, Halperin, Volgy, & Wissler, in press). Overall we have formulated five family therapy strategies: (1) developing and maintaining a therapeutic structure; (2) reality testing in the family; (3) interactional disengagement; (4) intervening in the intergenerational system; (5) solidification of the marital alliance and sibling subsystem.

The family therapist must evolve, from the outset, a carefully defined *therapeutic structure* that the family will experience as "safe." It is the therapeutic structure, which involves the processes of engaging the system and organizing the treatment, that provides a controlled setting and a safe milieu for the family. The issue of safety must be dealt with early because the intervention of the therapist often escalates the emotional intensity and apparent chaos of the system. The therapist must be sensitive to the system's vulnerability at the time of entering treatment.

The establishment of the structure is often pragmatic involving the agreements for time, day, frequency of appointments and who is to be present. While these initial steps define an outward structure they also set an underlying pattern of control by the therapist in essentially non-sensitive areas. The therapist who has difficulty setting limits or who cannot operationalize more than a "passive" therapeutic style will have great difficulty moving farther into therapy with borderline families.

We cannot overemphasize the importance of explicit rules of conduct in therapy in order to manage the inherent impulsivity of these systems and their occasional outbursts of violence. These dynamics must be anticipated because once they occur the therapist has already given up substantial control with a resultant loss of trust and power. The rules must be clear that threats, intimidation, or violence will not be tolerated in the therapy setting with the consequence that the person or persons involved will be asked to leave immediately. Therapy is defined for the family as a place where feelings and emotions will be examined and discussed but not acted upon. In our respective practices, we have seen too many cases where prior therapists failed to recognize the potential for violent escalation.

Once the structure has been established it must be maintained judiciously through the therapist's enforcement of rules, keeping appointments and being on time. Many therapists have discussed with us their personal reactivity to borderline families which often takes the form of covertly cancelling or being late for appointments. In one such case a therapist was delayed by an emergency in his office and sent word to the waiting borderline family that he would be another ten minutes. When he went to the reception area 20 minutes late to greet and apologize to the family they arose indignantly, shouted angry comments about his lack of interest in them, and knocked over a lamp as they rushed out of the office. They did not return to therapy.

The structure is maintained also by the therapist's appropriately timed expressions of caring and support. The structure is used by the therapist to carefully set the range of closeness and distance for each family system. As therapy progresses, the structure is gradually adjusted to allow the system to experience and tolerate more expressed conflict and distortions in a controlled manner without destructive consequences.

The borderline system's boundaries tend to be closed such that the family functions within its own narrowly constructed perception of reality that has been transposed across several generations. These closed boundaries not only serve to reinforce internal distortions but limit the therapist's early effort toward engagement and joining. Thus the therapist must represent a model a form of consensually validated external *reality* and bring this to bear on the perceptual and affective distortions of the system.

The distortions that can be recognized early by the therapist involve the interlocking processes of splitting and projective identification, erratic control swings within the parent-child subsystem, and a sense of collective despair. The therapist's role here is to join the system, experience with them their contextual distortions, and gradually challenge inaccurate perceptions and confirm more objective and functional data. Often gentle observations and humor go a long way in representing a new reality for the system.

At times the therapist will intervene to interrupt interactions so as to encourage members to "own" split off parts of themselves that have been projected onto others. The therapist will also use reframing where sensitive issues or dysfunctional behaviors are restated in such a manner that the family can accept the intervention without feeling too threatened. However, the therapist must be careful that the data of the reframe are basically congruent with the family's reality. Further distortions interjected into the system will often provoke withdrawal or chaotic reactions. Similarly, we would caution inexperienced therapists in the use of strategic and paradoxical techniques with borderline families. We have seen many cases where ill-conceived strategic interventions have provoked destructive acting-out or, at best, the perception of manipulation by the family.

As we have indicated, the borderline family's intensity and distortions are protected and maintained by a powerful symbiotic-like collusion among the members. The clinical task of *interactional disengagement* is conceived here as a process of creating and "marking" boundaries around both individual members and the respective subsystems. This moves toward the goal of actually restoring a level of expectable ambivalence to the interactions of the system so that members can begin to relate to one another as whole persons.

Frequently this will involve a direct challenge of the projective identification feedback loop between members by clear, pragmatic interventions. We have found that the use of video or audio tapes, played for the family from prior sessions, is useful in objectifying and diffusing these processes. The use of a co-therapy team facilitates this task in that it allows one therapist to enter the system and attempt to pull one member out of the projective loop while the other therapist remains outside of the system to provide stability and objectivity.

As we have reported, the intergenerational patterns of the borderline family are characterized by enmeshing loyalties and rigid structures which dysfunctionally bind one generation to the next. *Intergenerational interventions* and working with family of origin data serves to objectify and clarify historical issues and patterns as well as disengaging family members from repetitive historical dynamics. The inexperienced therapist should not view such work as merely the collection of genograms and social history data. Rather, intergenerational work should be seen as the weaving of a dramatic scenario by a master storyteller with the actual players and remnants of the system's rich history present in the office.

Typically, the therapist moves in and out of intergenerational data taking advantage of timing and the general flow and process of therapy. The decision to invite family of origin members into therapy must be based on their availability, the relative progress of therapy, and the degree of intrusion of such issues in present functioning. Again, inexperienced therapists must be cautious in deciding to bring such members into therapy with borderline families remembering that these figures may represent the source of primitive idealizations and projections. Often just the suggestion or preparation to bring in such members to therapy will trigger dramatic responses based on latent fear and apprehension. Frequently this is sufficient to move the therapy to a new level without ever bringing other members in. However, it is advised that the inclusion of family of origin members is best accomplished with a co-therapist present or with behind-the-mirror supervision or consultation available.

As these foregoing strategies begin to diffuse the interactional distortions, both internally and intergenerationally, it is possible to begin to mark and set new internal boundaries and renegotiate more clearly defined alliances within the parent-child subsystem. The clinical task of *solidifying the marital alliance and sibling subsystem* involves strengthening the boundaries of the spousal subsystem, reducing intergenerational loyalties of both spouses, and detriangling the "good" and "bad" children which will remove them from the spousal subsystem and return them to age-appropriate sibling roles.

The therapist should recall that the spousal and sibling subsystems, through their diffuse boundaries, are linked in circularly reinforcing roles. Thus to focus therapeutic attention on only one of these tasks would lead to the expectable sabotaging by the other subsystem. For example, the task of solidifying the marital alliance is dependent ont only on containing the persecuting child but also on removing the omnipotent child from the spousal subsystem. Underlying the accomplishment of these tasks is the probability that the removal of these triangles will quickly expose the vulnerabilities in the marital roles of the spouses.

These descriptive strategies are offered in a cursory manner to provide the family therapist with some guidelines for planning and monitoring family therapy treatment with borderline systems. They are expanded with further detail and illustrations elsewhere (Everett, Halperin, Volgy, and Wissler, in press). It is hoped that family therapists treating borderline families will perceive the critical linkage between careful assessment and the development of appropriate clinical strategies and will be able to further delineate these dimensions as such data accumulates in the field.

REFERENCES

APA (1980). *Diagnostic and Statistical Manual of Mental Disorders III, 2nd Ed.* Washington, DC.

Blanck, R. & Blanck, G. (1974). *Ego Psychology: Theory and Practice.* New York: Columbia University.

Bradley, S. J. (1981). The borderline diagnosis in children and adolescents. *Child Psychiatry and Human Development, 12,* 121-127.

Carter, L. & Rinsley, D. (1977). Vicissitudes of 'empathy' in a borderline adolescent. *International Review of Psycho-Analysis, 4,* 37-326.

Everett, C., Halperin, S., Volgy, S. & Wissler, A. (in press). The Borderline Family: Systemic Assessment and Treatment. New York: Grune & Stratton.

Grinker, R. & Werble, B. (1977). *The Borderline Patient.* New York: J. Aronson.

Gunderson, J. & Singer, M. (1975). Defining borderline patients: an overview. *American Journal of Psychiatry, 132,* 1-9.

Gunderson, J., Kerr, T. & England, D. (1980). The families of borderlines. *Archives of General Psychiatry, 37,* 27-33.

Guntrip, H. (1969). *Schizoid Phenomena, Object Relations and the Self.* New York: International University Press.

Jacobson, E. (1964). *The Self and the Object World.* New York: International University Press.

Kernberg, O. (1975). *Borderline Conditions and Pathological Narcissism.* New York: J. Aronson.

Kernberg, O. (1976). *Object Relations Theory and Clinical Psycho-Analysis.* New York: J. Aronson.

Mahler, M. (1971). A study of the separation-individuation process and its possible application to borderline phenomena in the psychoanalytic situation. *Psychoanalytic Study of the Child, 26,* 403-424.

Mahler, M., Pine, F. & Bergman, A. (1975). *The Psychological Birth of the Human Infant.* New York: Basic Books.

Masterson, J. & Rinsley, D. (1975). The borderline syndrome: the role of the mother in the genesis and psychic structure of the borderline personality. *International Journal of Psycho-Analysis, 56,* 163-177.

Nichols, W. & Everett, C. (1986). *Systemic Family Therapy: An Integrative Approach.* New York: Guilford Press.

Perry, J. & Klerman, G. (1978). The borderline patient. *Archives of General Psychiatry, 35,* 141-150.

Shapiro, E., Shapiro, R., Zinner, J. & Berkowitz, D. (1977). The borderline ego and the working alliance: indications for family and individual treatment in adolescence. *International Journal of Psycho-Analysis, 58,* 77-87.

Walsh, F. (1977). Family study 1976: 14 new borderline cases. In R. Grinker & B. Werble (Eds.), *The Borderline Patient.* New York: J. Aronson.

Zinner, J. & Shapiro, R. (1975). Splitting in families of borderline adolescents. In J. Mack (Ed.), *Borderline States in Psychiatry.* New York: Grune & Stratton.

Anxiety Disorders:
An Interactional View
of Agoraphobia

Michael Rohrbaugh
Glenn D. Shean

SUMMARY. Although biopsychiatry and learning theory continue to dominate thinking about anxiety disorders, there is growing evidence that marriage and family factors are profoundly relevant in the origin, maintenance, and successful treatment of the most common and chronically debilitating anxiety disorder, agoraphobia. It appears that (1) agoraphobia occurs in highly complementary, dominant-submissive relationships; (2) symptoms usually arise in response to real or anticipated changes in a vital relationship; (3) symptomatic improvement is often accompanied by increased marital conflict or the emergence of symptoms in a spouse; and (4) including the spouse as a co-therapist improves the outcome of treatment. These observations strain the linear, individualistic paradigms from which they have arisen. Interactional/ systems models of agoraphobia not only account for much of the current data, but have implications for treatment not derivable from competing paradigms.

Anxiety is a disease for the 1980s. According to a recent NIMH survey, an estimated 13.1 million Americans suffer from a DSM-III diagnosable anxiety disorder. The most common, chronically debilitating anxiety disorder is agoraphobia. Literally translated, agoraphobia means "fear of the market place" (Westphal, 1871). The chief complaint is fear of being away from a "safe" place or person, usually one's house or spouse. Incapacitating panic attacks and high levels of free-floating anxiety are common with agoraphobia, and normal activities are greatly restricted. The prevalence of this disorder in our

Michael Rohrbaugh and Glenn D. Shean are affiliated with College of William and Mary. Requests for reprints should be addressed to Michael Rohrbaugh, PhD, Department of Psychology, College of William and Mary, Williamsburg, VA 23185.

The authors are indebted to Joseph B. Eron for his contributions to an earlier draft of this paper.

65

society is high (.5% according to DSM-III) and apparently rising, with phobia clinics and self-help organizations proliferating across the country.

There is good evidence that both behavior therapy and drug therapy can be effective in reducing the intensity of agoraphobic symptoms. In fact, phobic disorders have been hailed as "psychotherapy's greatest success story" (Rosenhan & Seligman, 1984). Not surprisingly, the dominant theoretical models of agoraphobia are rooted in biopsychiatry and learning theory—paradigms which lead most clinicians to focus on the individual patient rather than the ecology of intimate relationships in which symptoms occur. From a family viewpoint, however, there are promising new developments: Researchers and clinicians are finding that the agoraphobic's current marriage and family relationships are profoundly relevant to understanding the course of this disorder and response to treatment. One purpose of this paper is to review these developments which, in our view, strain the linear, individualistic paradigms from which they have arisen. A second purpose is to recast existing observations and evidence into an interactional paradigm based on cybernetic and systems ideas (Watzlawick & Weakland, 1977; Hoffman, 1981; Rohrbaugh & Eron, 1982). We will propose that interactional models of agoraphobia not only account for much of the current data, but have implications for treatment not derivable from competing paradigms.

THE AGORAPHOBIC SYNDROME

The chief complaint in agoraphobia is a fear of leaving home. Most agoraphobics are not able to venture outside the home unless accompanied by a trusted person. Patients typically fear being in public, open, or crowded places, and sometimes cannot be alone at home. DSM-III distinguishes two subtypes of the disorder based on the presence or absence of panic attacks (which has implications for chemotherapy). Panic attacks reportedly "come out of the blue." In fact, some researchers believe that a fear of losing control, or "fear of fear" (Goldstein & Chambless, 1978), is central to the disorder. Agoraphobia commonly occurs with other problems such as depression, sexual dysfunction, hypochondriacal concerns, transient episodes of depersonalization, and family conflict (Chambless, 1982).

Agoraphobic symptoms typically follow a fluctuating course, with periods of relative freedom interspersed with longer periods of severe incapacitation. Although some patients "spontaneously" recover (Agras, Chapin & Oliveau, 1972), the disorder is often chronic and symptoms can last a lifetime. The mean age of onset is 28 years (Burns & Thorpe, 1977) and symptoms typically begin following a period of transition and interpersonal stress. Unlike other phobias which appear to distribute equally across sexes, the vast majority of diagnosed agoraphobics are married women (Vandereycken, 1983). Surveys suggest that females comprise 75% (Agras, Sylvester & Oliveau, 1969) to 95% (Marks & Herse, 1970) of this population. Since few agoraphobics hold jobs outside the home (Burns & Thorpe, 1977), the disorder is sometimes called "housewife's disease."

THEORY DETERMINES WHAT WE SEE . . .

Despite general agreement on the clinical picture in agoraphobia, theoretical formulations vary widely. It is difficult to overestimate the extent to which the paradigmatic lens through which we view a disorder influences what we pay attention to and what we do not. As Watzlawick (1974) notes, paraphrasing Einstein, "the theory determines what we see in therapy" – and ultimately what we do. This is especially important when it comes to the family since the more established psychodynamic, biological and behavioral paradigms constrain how we think about family interaction, and sometimes distract attention from it entirely. From an interactional perspective, it is constraining to assume that agoraphobia is a disorder of one person.

The psychoanalytic view (Freud, 1932) is that agoraphobia is an expression of dependency needs (Bowlby, 1973) or deep-seated unconscious conflicts rooted in the past (Freud, 1932). In either case, the current marital or family environment is not emphasized. An important prediction from psychodynamic theory is that new problems will emerge if phobic symptoms are removed precipitously, without addressing the underlying intrapsychic cause. As we will see, there is evidence that new symptoms often *do* appear following rapid symptom removal (Milton & Hafner, 1979; Hafner, 1984). The fact that they often appear in people other than the identified patient, however, suggests that interactional as well as intrapsychic processes may be involved.

In the current psychiatric mainstream, the psychodynamic view has taken a back seat to biological psychiatry as a framework for understanding agoraphobia. According to the biological paradigm, agoraphobia, or "anxiety disease," is caused by a genetically determined vulnerability to "endogenous anxiety" (Sheehan, 1982, 1983; Theyer, Neese, Cameron & Curtis, 1985) or "separation anxiety" (Liebowitz & Klein, 1983). Panic attacks have been linked to vestibular abnormalities (Jacobs, Miller, Turner & Wall, 1985), sensitivity to caffeine (Charney, Heninger & Jatlow, 1985), and physiological problems such as mitral valve prolapse. Supporting evidence for the biological view comes from research indicating that antidepressant medications can be effective in controlling the "spontaneous" panic attacks assumed to be the core of the agoraphobic syndrome (Sheehan, 1983). While allowing that the family may be relevant as a gene pool, proponents of the biological view have paid little attention to the marital or family context of agoraphobia in their theoretical explanations and therapeutic interventions. We should note, however, that biological premises do not preclude a possible role for family interaction in the maintenance or exacerbation of agoraphobic symptoms. In fact, a stress-diathesis model similar to that which provides a framework for the "psychoeducational" treatments of schizophrenia (Anderson, Hogarty & Reiss, 1980; Falloon, Boyd & McGill, 1984) might as readily be applied here. In this formulation, family interaction is a potential stress factor which, when combined with the patient's constitutional vulnerability, can cause "anxiety disease."

Behavioral models of agoraphobia based on learning theory are supported by an even larger body of research, including many clinical outcome studies (Emmelkamp, 1982; Goldstein, 1982; Marks, 1981; Mathews, 1981). As might be expected, behaviorists criticize the long-term treatment of agoraphobia with pharmacotherapy alone (Telch et al., 1983) and offer their own evidence that behavior therapy is at least as effective as drug therapy (Michelson & Mavissikalian, 1985).

Behavioral models assume that the disorder is acquired through Pavlovian conditioning, avoidance conditioning, and cognitive learning. Anxiety and panic come to be elicited by a variety of exteroceptive and interoceptive cues, either by virtue of their association with some real or imagined trauma, or through vicarious learning. Fear and panic responses generalize rapidly to other stimuli, mobilizing a range of instrumental avoidance behaviors (agoraphobia) which are reinforced by anxiety reduction. Avoidance behavior, in turn, is self-perpetuating because it prevents the patient from coming into contact with anxiety arousing stimuli so that extinction can occur. Cognitive-behaviorists add that irrational beliefs and cognitive distortions also play a role in maintaining symptoms (Beck, Laude & Bohnert, 1974; Emmelkamp & Mersch, 1982).

The main treatment principle which follows from learning models is *exposure*. In one way or another—gradually or precipitously, through assignments that clients carry out in imagination or in vivo, either alone or in the company of a trusted other—the therapist arranges for the patient to face the feared situation until extinction of conditioned anxiety responses can occur. Whatever the procedural specifics, exposure strategies are commonly used in conjunction with other interventions such as relaxation training, breathing exercises, cognitive reorientation, assertiveness training, social skills training, and conjoint marital therapy (Goldstein, 1982; Emmelkamp, 1982; Mathews, Gelder & Johnston, 1981). When marital therapy is used, it is viewed as an adjunctive intervention for co-existing marital problems which may complicate the clinical picture, but are distinct from the agoraphobia per se (Cobb, McDonald, Marks & Stern, 1980).

Research has consistently shown that exposure-based behavioral treatments compare favorably to a variety of control procedures. Although some authorities conclude that phobias have been virtually conquered (Rosenhan & Seligman, 1984), others acknowledge that currently available treatments are not perfect. In a review of outcome research, Barlow and Mavissikalian (1981) point out that while 60-75% of treated phobics improve, only 4-18% become totally symptom free. These statistics, furthermore, are based only on patients who complete treatment; yet agoraphobic patients are notorious for dropping out of therapy, with attrition rates in some studies approaching 30%. Seen in this light, published outcome data are less impressive since barely half of the agoraphobics treated in research settings may be getting better. To complicate the outcome question further, there are reports that exposure therapies may be less effective for male agoraphobics than for females (Guidano & Liotti, 1976). In any case, for a variety of reasons, it is probably premature to conclude that the therapeutic book on agoraphobia has been closed.

Given the paradigmatic constraints mentioned above, it is surprising how much attention the literature on agoraphobia gives to factors *other* than the individual patient's symptoms. It has been repeatedly observed, for example, that the disorder occurs in highly complementary, dominant-submissive relationships (Fodor, 1974; Hafner, 1984); that married patients show an exaggerated dependence on a "well" spouse who appears to be reinforced by this dependence (Agulnik, 1970; Bergner, 1977); and that symptomatic improvement is often accompanied by increased marital conflict or the appearance of symptoms in the spouse (Milton & Hafner, 1979; Hafner, 1984). Some behavior therapists suggest that the agoraphobic syndrome may *only* occur in patients who feel trapped in a difficult interpersonal relationship (Goldstein & Chambless, 1981). Others recommend that the spouse routinely be included in exposure treatment as a co-therapist

(Vandereycken, 1983; Hafner, 1984), and for some couples at least, this appears to improve outcome (Barlow, O'Brien & Last, 1984; Cobb, Mathews, Childs-Clarke & Blowers, 1984).

In the next section, we will outline four empirically-supported propositions about the family context of agoraphobia. Although the supporting data have arisen largely from the behavioral paradigm, they also fit well with an interactional/systems view.

AGORAPHOBIA AND THE FAMILY

1. *Agoraphobia occurs in highly complementary relationships, particularly marriages organized according to traditional sex roles.*

Almost by definition, agoraphobics are highly dependent on another person, usually a spouse. For over 30 years, clinicians have noted distinctive features of the agoraphobic's marriage. In an early study comparing 25 female agoraphobics to patients with conversion hysteria and anxiety neurosis, Webster (1953) suggested that phobic symptoms may be part of a mutual caretaking strategy in which the wife's dependency needs are met by the husband who in turn is helped to feel competent and to ignore his own problems. Tucker (1956) noted that husbands assume the role of father in the agoraphobic marriage. Agulnik (1970) later observed that agoraphobic patients are extremely dependent on a spouse who appears to be "spuriously fortified" by this dependence. He proposed that "assortative mating" occurs, at least in some agoraphobic marriages. Similarly, Goodstein and Swift (1977) hypothesized that agoraphobics seek the "ideal parent" in a marriage partner, and Bergner (1977) suggested that partners marry hoping to find attributes in their spouses that are lacking in themselves.

These observations suggest that agoraphobia is associated with highly *complementary* rather than symmetrical relationships, (Bateson, 1972). In other words, symptoms occur in an interactional context characterized by exchanges of opposite behavior (dominance-submission, helplessness-nurturance) rather than similar behavior or equal behavior. Thus, Fodor (1974) observed that agoraphobic women exhibit an extreme stereotype of female behavior and tend to choose men who complement their helplessness, dependency, and lack of assertiveness by exhibiting the extremes of the male sex role stereotype.

Beyond the issue of dependency, the complementarity in agoraphobic relationships can take different forms. Hafner (1977), for example, found two marital sub-types among female patients based on questionnaire measures of hostility and intro-extropunitiveness: In one, the patient was hostile and extropunitive and the spouse was intropunitive; in the other, the pattern was reversed. Liotti and Guidano (1976) described a somewhat different kind of marital complementarity in a sample of 15 male agoraphobics. Here, the patients were socially extraverted, ambitious, and assertive, at least before the symptoms began. However, they were unable to communicate intimate emotions directly, and required reassurance from the wife about their health concerns. The wives, on the other hand, tended to be introverted and socially anxious. They were able to be calm and reassuring in dealings with the husband but expected him to be outgoing and provide a pleasant social life in return.

In the relatively infrequent cases where agoraphobia occurs outside of a marriage, interaction around the symptoms is also highly complementary. In our own work, we have seen young-adult agoraphobics whose main attachment was to a parent, and other patients who, while unmarried, were enmeshed in highly restrictive marriage-like relationships. Goldstein (1982) and Guidano and Liotti (1983) note similar cases in which unmarried agoraphobics were in ongoing, conflictually dependent relationships with their families of origin. Goldstein (1982), for example, described a situation in which a mother and daughter were *both* agoraphobic. Their symptoms followed an alternating, complementary pattern in which one person would be relatively symptom free when the other was most incapacitated.

2. Close relatives of agoraphobics, particularly their spouses, often have problems too.

Many of the clinical reports cited above also make reference to apparent dysfunction of the patient's spouse or another family member. Husbands of agoraphobic women, for example, have been variously described as rigid, detached, jealous, insecure, sexually inadequate, and generally neurotic (Fry, 1962; Bergner, 1977; Goodstein & Swift, 1977; Hafner, 1970; Quadrio, 1983). Evidence from studies employing more systematic, objective measures of spouse functioning is limited and not entirely consistent. Agulnik (1970) based his assortative mating hypothesis on high correlations between the neuroticism scores of spouses and agoraphobic patients married less than ten years. On the other hand, Buglass, Clarke, Henderson, Kreitman, and Presley (1977), using self-report measures, found few differences between the husbands of 30 agoraphobics and those of matched controls. Hafner (1982), however, has criticized the conclusions of Buglass et al. in some detail, suggesting that they overlooked evidence of dissimulation by husbands of the agoraphobics.

3. Agoraphobic symptoms arise in response to real or anticipated changes in a vital relationship (or relationships) and function to pre-serve former patterns.

There is evidence that the onset of agoraphobia correlates with ac-tual or portended shifts in intimate relationships, some of which are inevitable in the family life cycle. Generalizing from a sample of ago-raphobics studied in Italy, Guidano and Liotti (1983) reported that initial symptoms commonly occurred (1) just before or shortly follow-ing a marriage; (2) when the patient is about to leave home or become more independent of his or her parents; (3) when new affective rela-tionships were being formed outside the family; (4) after important life events such as a loss, the birth of a child, or a change in work activity that makes one partner more or less independent than before; or (5) during a marital crisis when one partner makes a move toward separa-tion. Essentially similar observations have been made by Goldstein (1970) and Goldstein and Chambless (1978), who note that symptoms usually arise in a climate of interpersonal conflict over a seemingly unresolvable issue — often when someone wants to change a relation-ship.

The intriguing aspect is that symptom onset usually *forestalls* rela-tionship change, having the effect of preserving complementary inter-action patterns, but in an unsatisfactory way. Liotti and Guidano's (1976) description of symptom development in male agoraphobics provides a vivid illustration:

> Before the appearance of the husband's neurotic disturbance, aggressive interchanges between partners were rare, mainly be-cause the wife seemed to have accepted a submissive position. During a period immediately preceding the appearance of the husband's symptoms there was a sharp rise in the frequency of marital quarrels. Most often this appeared to be precipitated by the wife's departure from the original contract, and in particular a move away from marital submission. This movement was followed by marital quarreling and the typical reaction of the wife to the husband's (usually verbal) aggression was either ex-aggerated anxiety reaction or a prompt emotional withdrawal fol-lowed by a period of resentful silence. With the onset of the husband's neurotic fears the marital quarrels showed a reduction in intensity and reverted to a series of continuous, monotonous arguments . . .
>
> Ultimately a new reinforcement contract between husband and wife emerges based on a somewhat paradoxical rule regarding dominance and submission. The husband is given the opportu-

nity to assert himself and dominate his wife by deciding what actions are possible or not—this being determined very largely by the likelihood of his having an anxiety attack. At the same time the wife can feel she is really the dominant partner because she is not being obedient but rather assisting him in a way that one might assist a sick or childish person. (p. 162)

4. *Symptomatic improvement may have negative repercussions in the family system.*

The idea that symptoms provide interpersonal benefits or "secondary gains" for the patient is not new. Most interactional formulations of agoraphobia, on the other hand, emphasize the adaptive or protective function of symptoms for either the spouse or for the stability of the marital relationship itself (Vandereycken, 1983; Fry, 1962).

One way to determine if agoraphobic symptoms serve an adaptive function for a family is to observe the consequences of their removal. Again, most relevant observations concern the agoraphobic marriage: Spouses sometimes sabotage treatment (Emmelkamp, 1974; Hafner, 1982), and symptomatic improvement is often accompanied by marital discord (Goodstein & Swift, 1977; Hand & Lamontagne, 1976; Milton & Hafner, 1979) or by the emergence of symptoms in the spouse (Milton & Hafner, 1979; Hafner, 1984).

Of particular interest is a series of studies undertaken by Hafner and his associates in England (Hafner, 1976; Milton & Hafner, 1979) and continued in Australia (Hafner, 1982, 1984). Hafner found that changes in agoraphobic symptoms during and following intensive (one to two week) exposure therapy correlated with changes in the quality of the patients' marital relationships and levels of distress reported by their husbands. In one cohort (Hafner, 1976), the husbands of 33 patients showed increased "neuroticism" as treatment progressed, concomitant with improvement in their wives' symptoms. Later, when some of the wives relapsed, their husbands reportedly improved. In a partial replication of this study (Milton & Hafner, 1979), nine of 18 marriages appeared to be adversely affected by symptomatic improvement in the identified patient. Furthermore, patients with the worst marriages (according to a marital satisfaction inventory) improved least and were most likely to relapse in the six months following therapy. This last finding has been confirmed by Bland and Hallam (1981), who found that marital satisfaction measured before therapy predicted outcome of exposure treatment at six-month follow-up.

From a more recent one-year follow-up of 32 agoraphobic women, Hafner (1984) reports several distinct patterns of marital response to rapid improvement in the wives' symptoms following exposure treatment. Eighteen of the couples showed increased competition and marital conflict about autonomy and sex role expectations (such as whether the wife would work outside the home), and the husbands in 12 of these couples developed psychological symptoms which effectively slowed the wife's progress in the first half of the follow-up period. By the one-year follow-up, however, the marital systems of most of these couples had largely adapted, with both partners achieving more autonomy, and the wives' maintaining their symptomatic gains. In the second pattern, couples continued in rigidly complementary (dominant-submissive) interactions. Overt marital conflict was minimal in the first half of the follow-up period, but increased dramatically thereafter. For these couples, Hafner hypothesized that continuing symptomatic improvement at one year depended on the couple's success in resolving these sex-role issues.

5. *Including the spouse as a co-therapist improves treatment outcome.*

Although some of Hafner's conclusions have been questioned (Marks, 1981; Emmelkamp & van der Hout, 1982), many behavior therapists now acknowledge the importance of marital dynamics in agoraphobia and recommend including the spouse in treatment. In a recent literature review, Vandereycken (1983) concluded that, whenever possible, exposure treatment should involve the spouse as a co-therapist from the very beginning. The advantages cited include: not alienating the spouse, who can easily undermine treatment (Hafner, 1982); helping the spouse accept and positively reinforce changes in the patient's behavior (Mathews, Teasdale et al., 1977; Benjamin & Kincey, 1977; Chambless & Goldstein, 1981); enlisting the spouse's aid in carrying out specific therapeutic tasks (Barlow, Mavissikalian & Hay, 1981; Mathews et al., 1981); helping the spouse acknowledge his own problems (Hafner, 1982); and being in a position to address marital issues when they arise (Vandereycken, 1983; Hand, Spoehring & Stanik, 1977; Hafner, 1982). Many of the same authors are also sensitive to the *manner* in which the spouse is included in treatment. In interactional terms, they respect the rigid complementarity of the patient's marriage by defining the spouse not as "co-patient" (which "marriage therapy" would imply) but as "co-therapist." In fact, Hand et al. (1977) have discussed the usefulness of "hidden couple-counseling" with some cases: In effect, the therapist does behavioral marital therapy without calling it such, subtly shifting the focus of tasks and suggestions through the course of treatment from the patient's fears to the husband and wife's interaction.

Several recent experimental studies confirm that including the spouse as a co-therapist can indeed improve the outcome of behavioral treatment (Barlow, O'Brien & Last, 1984; Cobb, Mathews, Childe-Clarke & Blowers, 1984). Barlow et al. found that women patients treated with their husbands showed substantially better symptomatic improvement than women treated without their husbands. There were similar differences between the groups in social and family functioning during treatment, but these disappeared by follow-up. Unlike the intensive ("drag 'em kicking and screaming to the mall") exposure used in the British studies, Barlow's procedure allowed patients to undertake exposure at their own pace over a 12-week period. Weekly group meetings followed an educational format in which therapists taught cognitive mastery techniques, relaxation skills, etc., which patients were encouraged to use in self-initiated exposure trials. In contrast to Hafner's studies, symptomatic improvement was not associated with deterioration in the marriage, a finding which the authors attributed to the gradual pacing of their treatment regime. Most interesting, however, were comparisons of patients who improved and those who did not based on daily logs kept by the subjects. The researchers expected to find that the patients who improved had practiced more, due to receiving increased encouragement and support from their husbands. They found instead that the compliance and practice patterns of successful and unsuccessful patients were roughly comparable — yet the husbands of those who improved felt better able to understand and deal with their wives' fears. The implication is that exposure per se may have had less to do with patients overcoming their fears than changes that occurred in their marriages.

Data such as Hafner's and Barlow's seem to strain the linear, individualistic paradigm of learning theory in which most family studies of agoraphobia have been conducted. If agoraphobia is localized in one person and understood as a learned avoidance response maintained by anxiety reduction, clinical procedures based on extinguishing fear by exposing the patient to what she is afraid of make good sense. But interactional phenomena are then split off as stress factors, motivating conditions, or sources of secondary gain — and the marriage or family is important only insofar as it complicates or obstructs the treatment process. From an interactional perspective, this kind of dualistic (and artificial) separation of symptom and system is misleading and unnecessary. By formulating the problem in terms of ongoing circular interaction patterns which both maintain and are maintained by the symptom, the unit of analysis and intervention expands and becomes more flexible, encompassing not only the patient's own self-defeating attempts to solve the problem, but the rule-governed structure of the marriage (or family) relationship itself.

TOWARD AN INTERACTIONAL VIEW

The "interactional view," which many regard as the ideological core of the family therapy movement, has its roots in Gregory Bateson's (1952-62) research project on communication (Watzlawick & Weakland, 1977; Haley, 1981; Hoffman, 1981). Psychiatrist William Fry (1962), a member of the original Bateson group, published a rich description of "the marital context of an anxiety syndrome" in the first volume of *Family Process*. Fry began by observing that agoraphobic symptoms in a series of cases he had seen were intimately related to the patient's marital situation, noting that on close examination the "well" spouse (mostly husbands) revealed a history of symptoms closely resembling those of the wife. The patient's symptoms, furthermore, appeared to protect the spouse, who in turn tended to be highly protective of the patient (e.g., phoning regularly, staying home, offering reassurance when it wasn't requested). In each case, the onset of symptoms coincided with an important and potentially threatening change in the life of the spouse. Once established, the symptoms served to "support the continuing functioning of the spouse" and "maintain the marriage at times when it threatened to break up." Fry termed these marriages "compulsory" because they were maintained by elaborate systems of "dual control" which tied both partners down while keeping them united in a difficult and conflictual relationship. Years later, in describing marriages which deteriorated in the British behavior therapy studies, Milton and Hafner (1979) cited two patterns which directly parallel Fry's observations:

> In one pattern, the patient's symptoms appeared to strengthen aspects of largely affectionless "compulsory" marriages; in the other, the patient's symptoms appeared to protect their spouses from recognizing or examining aspects of their own personal and interpersonal problems. (p. 807)

The interactional view is based mainly on cybernetics and systems theory. A key assumption is that regardless of how problems originate, they persist as aspects of current, ongoing interaction systems. Cybernetic feedback processes provide a framework for understanding how symptoms are *maintained*, which is of greater interest than etiological hypotheses or linear (historical) notions of cause and effect. It is further assumed that problems occur not so much within people as between them — that psychological "symptoms" and interaction systems are inextricably interwoven. Thus, the interactional paradigm offers a fundamentally different view of what agoraphobia *is*. The patient's fear of leaving home is less an abnormality of one person than an element in a recursive interaction process which inevitably requires several people for its maintenance. As Lazarus, the behaviorist, put it 20 years ago: "It is presumably impossible to become an agoraphobic without the aid of someone who will submit to the inevitable demands imposed upon them by the sufferer" (1966, p. 97).

The interactional/systems paradigm has evolved in different directions since the Bateson project and the publication of Fry's paper. Most noteworthy was the emergence of distinct yet related family therapy models based on interactional premises (Weakland, Fisch, Watzlawick & Bodin, 1974; Haley, 1976, 1980; Minuchin, 1974; Selvini Palazzoli, Boscolo, Cecchin & Prata, 1978; Hoffman, 1981). All of these models are "systemic" in their allegiance to ecological, cybernetic formulations of problem maintenance. Most are also "strategic," in that the therapist intervenes deliberately, on the basis of a specific plan, to resolve the presenting problem as efficiently as possible. Depending on the model, intervention might involve interdicting problem-maintaining interaction cycles or restructuring the relationships with which the symptom is interwoven. Change is not assumed to depend on insight, education, emotional release, or the acquisition of problem-solving skills. Although the therapist may "reframe" the meaning of events or behavior, the purpose is not to provide insight, but to provoke change. If the problem can be solved without clients knowing how or why, that is satisfactory (Madanes, 1981).

In the cybernetic framework of the strategic systems therapies, there are at least two different ways to understand the interactional maintenance of agoraphobic symptoms. One we will call a *functional/structural* formulation and the other an *accidental/sequential* formulation. The "functionalist" view, based on a negative feedback model, assumes that symptoms serve a stabilizing function for either another family member (the spouse) or for the family (marriage) itself. The symptom is also assumed to maintain (as it is maintained by) the relationship "structure" in which it occurs. In contrast, the "accidentalist" view[1] focuses on the (mostly dyadic) interaction sequences in which symptoms are embedded. The model of problem maintenance is a simple positive feedback loop, or vicious cycle. It is not assumed that the symptom serves a function for the family or its members: problem-maintaining sequences simply happen — as if by accident.

Functional/Structural Formulations

Negative feedback formulations are central to the theories of Haley (1976), Minuchin (1974), Hoffman (1981) and others. They "explain" how systems maintain their equilibrium or stability. In error-activated fashion, increases in one variable are linked to decreases in another, keeping some key system parameter within tolerable limits. Thus, increasing symptoms in one spouse may be associated with decreasing distress in the other. Or, the homeostatic variable could be a property of the marriage itself—for example, the balance of power or caretaking functions between the spouses, or the level of conflict or aggression they express. When the agoraphobic's highly complementary, dominant-submissive marriage shifts toward symmetry (as when the submissive spouse becomes more assertive or the dominant spouse falters), the appearance of symptoms may restore the former balance, though usually in a conflictual and unsatisfactory way. This formulation is essentially consistent with the clinical observations and research findings discussed above (e.g., Liotti & Guidano, 1976; Hafner, 1982, 1984).

At a dyadic level, therapy based on the functional/structural idea attempts to shift the complementary relationship structure toward symmetry and disentangle fear symptoms from their hypothesized protective functions. An important strategic principle is to avoid challenging the problematic relationship directly—even when working to change it. At the beginning of treatment it may be especially counterproductive, as Hafner (1982), Vandereycken (1983) and others point out, to suggest that the patient's fears may reflect marital problems or that marital therapy is indicated. A better strategy is to request that the spouse participate because he or she is an essential resource, knowing more about the problem than anyone outside the family. (Defining the spouse as "co-therapist" fits very well with this idea.) When the wife is the patient, a useful joining tactic is to support the husband's executive position in the dyad, at least initially, by seeing him alone and/or asking his advice about certain aspects of the wife's treatment. When the husband is the patient, respecting and working with complementarity can be more difficult because the power hierarchy (dominant husband as patient, submissive wife as caretaker) is more incongruously defined (Madanes, 1981).

Respecting complementarity is equally important when the therapist attempts to intervene more directly. The overtly dominant spouse should be consulted about, and if possible put in charge of, homework assignments. For example, when exposure is prescribed, the husband can be asked to monitor the wife's progress closely, allowing her to go no further than he feels she can tolerate—the assumption being that she would go no further than he, or they, could tolerate anyway (Haley, 1976). The therapist can sometimes facilitate progress along these lines by using gentle restraining tactics, such as worrying vaguely about other problems that might arise if the patient overcomes her fears (Fisch, Weakland & Segal, 1982). In some cases it is possible to shift a couple toward symmetry by exaggerating or pushing their complementarity to an extreme. If the "well" spouse is asked to take over *all* executive functions, and the patient not to venture even so far as the garden without the spouse's permission, the couple may rebel by reorganizing in a more symmetrical way (Hoffman, 1981; Madanes, 1981).

In these approaches, the conceptual unit is the dyad. Yet with other problems, structural/functional family therapy theories emphasize interaction patterns at the level of the triad. It is not difficult to imagine how agoraphobic symptoms could stabilize relationships beyond a dyad. For example, the patient's intense involvement with one parent may maintain (and be maintained by) a distant or conflictual relationship between that parent and the other parent. Or the agoraphobic may align with a parent (or child, or therapist) against his or her spouse. In the triadic view, symptomatic dysfunction reflects dominant alliances and coalitions that cross generation lines (Haley, 1980; Hoffman, 1981). There is little direct evidence linking these kinds of triadic patterns to agoraphobia, but in our experience they are common. Solyom, Silberfeld and Solyom (1976) did find a high frequency of "overprotective reactions" in the mothers of adult agoraphobics, and Goldstein (1982) has noted that many female agoraphobics maintain a "primary attachment" with their mother. Goldstein adds that these are the most difficult cases to treat. Due to paradigm constraints, it is not surprising that behavioral clinicians do not view such intense cross-generational ties in the context of broader triadic patterns of dysfunction. In general, interventions based on such a triadic formulation of problem maintenance would attempt to weaken cross-generational coalitions while strengthening intra-generational ties (Minuchin, 1974). This would usually require including several generations in therapy. In some cases, the therapist might even put the parent generation in charge of the patient's fears, following Haley's (1980) approach to treating "leaving home" problems.

Accidental/Sequential Formulations

The leading "accidentalist" model is the interactional view of problem maintenance developed by Fisch, Weakland, Watzlawick and others at the Mental Research Institute in Palo Alto (Weakland et al., 1974; Fisch et al., 1982). Unlike "functionalist" approaches based on the negative feedback model, the Palo Alto vision of problem maintenance is a simple positive feedback loop centering around well-intentioned but inappropriate "solutions." Here, "more of the same" solution leads to more of the problem, leading to more solution, and so on, in an ever-escalating vicious cycle. The assumption is that problems would be self-limiting were it not for the persistent but misguided problem-solving attempts of the people involved. Theoretical constructions about the "functions" of symptoms and the "structure" of relationships are not relevant since the focus is restricted to solution behaviors which directly impinge upon the problem. In this view, the problem *is* the solution, and interdicting the solution, even in a small way, paves the way for change (Watzlawick et al., 1974).

In a dyadic analysis using this model, attention focuses on the specific, highly repetitive interaction sequences which the patient and his or her helpers engage in around the symptoms. In agoraphobia, oscillating patterns of reassurance, overprotection, hypervigilance or withdrawal often interlock with the symptoms – and any of these patterns could be a target for strategic intervention. The goal would be to persuade the spouse(s) to do *less* of the same, using whatever rationale he or she (or they) would be likely to accept. The spouse who does too much for the patient would be asked to do too little, the spouse who encourages might be asked to be gently discouraging, and so on. With male agoraphobics especially, it can be helpful to arrange that husband and wife simply not talk about the problem with each other, except at prescribed times and places, such as the therapist's office. When mindreading or hypervigilance by the spouse is an issue, the interactional circuits may be "jammed" by asking the patient to *pretend* to be anxious (or not anxious) and the spouse to try to ascertain, without commenting, whether she is really feeling that way. (This also requires a plausible rationale such as helping the spouse increase his or her sensitivity to the patient's symptoms.) Even if the patient fails to comply with the directive to pretend, the jamming intervention may introduce enough uncertainty to disrupt the usual interaction pattern (Fisch et al., 1982).

The problem-maintaining solution principle applies equally to the patient's own struggle with the problem. With agoraphobia, this presents a curious theoretical reversal: while individually-oriented behavior therapists have been discovering the importance of interaction, the Palo Alto interactionists have been acknowledging "self-referential" aspects of anxiety disorders. According to Fisch et al. (1982),

. . . anxiety states can arise and be maintained without help from anyone else. This does not mean that others do not aid in maintaining such problems; often they do. We simply mean that these kinds of problems do not need such "help" in order to occur and persist. (pp. 136-137)

Fisch et al. go on to suggest that, in anxiety problems, the patient's problem-maintaining attempted solution is to avoid the feared task while pushing herself or himself to master it. The thrust of intervention, therefore, is to "expose the patient to the task while restraining him from completing it." Note that at the individual level this approach generates an intervention strategy which, in principle, closely resembles the exposure treatments derived from learning theory. In practice, however, the techniques for effecting exposure can be quite different (Fisch et al., 1982, pp. 137-139).

CONCLUSION

There can be little doubt that family interaction is profoundly related to the agoraphobic syndrome, yet how best to understand that relationship will be a subject of continuing controversy. In our view, interactional models of the disorder not only fit the clinical and research data as well or better than competing paradigms, but also suggest additional guidelines for intervention. But others will surely disagree (Cobb et al., 1980; Mathews et al., 1981; Burns & Thorpe, 1977). It is unlikely that such paradigmatic issues will soon be resolved by empirical research. In fact, the many claims and counterclaims about findings in this area are reminiscent of Kuhn's (1962) comments on the limits to communication between proponents of different paradigms, and the difference between what each takes to be facts.

Within the interactional paradigm, important issues remain. As our discussion of "functionalist" and "accidentalist" approaches to agoraphobia illustrates, an interactional view can be applied at several system levels, including the level of the individual. In addition, system levels beyond the natural family may be relevant, as when a patient seeks help from several professionals at the same time or participates in a self-help group against the spouse's wishes. Even within a consistent theoretical framework, therapists must address the question of which level(s) of system—individual, patient-family, or helper-patient-family—have priority for intervention under what circumstances. When problem patterns are identified at several of these levels simultaneously, where is the best place to intervene? An implication of the interactional/systems view is that expanding the conceptual problem unit will be fruitful clinically.

Finally, the fact that interactional factors are important in agoraphobia does not mean that they are equally important in other anxiety syndromes such as post-traumatic stress disorder, panic disorder, generalized anxiety disorder, social/simple phobia, or obsessive-compulsive disorder. With but a few exceptions (e.g., Hoover & Insel, 1984), studies of non-agoraphobic anxiety problems have paid surprisingly little attention to family interaction.

NOTE

1. The term "accidentalism" was introduced by Jeffrey Bogdan in a panel presentation at the Family Therapy Network Symposium, Washington, DC, March, 1985.

REFERENCES

Agras, W. S., Sylvester, D., & Oliveau, D. (1969). The epidemiology of common fears and phobias. *Comprehensive Psychiatry, 10,* 151-156.

Agras, W. S., Chapin, H. N., & Oliveau, D. C. (1972). The natural history of phobia. *Archives of General Psychiatry, 26,* 315-317.

Agulnik, P. L. (1970). The spouse of the phobic patient. *British Journal of Psychiatry, 117,* 59-67.

Anderson, C. H., Hogarty, G., & Reiss, D. J. (1980). Family treatment of adult schizophrenic patients: A psychoeducational approach. *Schizophrenia Bulletin, 6,* 490-505.

Barlow, D. H., & Mavissikalian, M. (1981). Directions in the assessment and treatment of phobia: The next decade. In M. Mavissikalian & D. H. Barlow (Eds.), *Phobia: Psychological and pharmacological treatment.* New York: Guilford Press.

Barlow, D. H., Mavissikalian, M., & Hay, L. R. (1981). Couples treatment of agoraphobia: Changes in marital satisfaction. *Behaviour Research and Therapy, 19,* 245-255.

Barlow, D. H., O'Brien, G. T., & Last, C. G. (1984). Couples treatment of agoraphobia. *Behavior Therapy, 16,* 41-58.

Bateson, G. (1972). *Steps to an ecology of mind.* New York: Random House.

Beck, A. T., Laude, R., & Bohnert, M. (1974). Ideational components of anxiety neurosis. *Archives of General Psychiatry, 31,* 319-325.

Bergner, R. M. (1977). The marital system of the hysterical individual. *Family Process, 16,* 85-96.

Bland, K., & Hallam, R. S. (1981). Relationship between response to graded exposure and marital satisfaction in agoraphobics. *Behaviour Research and Therapy, 19,* 335-338.

Bowlby, J. (1973). *Attachment and loss. Vol. 2. Separation*. London: Hogarth Press.

Buglass, D., Clarke, J., Henderson, A. S., Kreitman, N., & Presley, A. S. (1977). A study of agoraphobic housewives. *Psychological Medicine, 7*, 73-86.

Burns, L. E., & Thorpe, G. L. (1977). Fears and clinical phobias: Epidemiological aspects and the national survey of agoraphobics. *Journal of International Medical Research, 5* (Suppl. I), 132-139.

Chambless, D. (1982). Characteristics of agoraphobics. In D. L. Chambless & A. J. Goldstein (Eds.), *Agoraphobia: Multiple perspectives on theory and treatment*. New York: Wiley & Sons.

Chambless, D. L., & Goldstein, A. J., Eds. (1982). *Agoraphobia: Multiple perspectives on theory and treatment*. New York: Wiley & Sons.

Chambless, D. L., & Goldstein, A. J. (1981). Clinical treatment of agoraphobia. In M. Mavissikalian & D. H. Barlow (Eds.). *Phobia: Psychological and pharmacological treatment*. New York: Guilford Press, 1981.

Charney, D., & Heninger, G. (1985). Increased anxiogenic effects of caffeine in panic disorders. *Archives of General Psychiatry, 42*, 233-243.

Cobb, J., McDonald, R., Marks, I., & Stern, R. (1980). Marital versus exposure therapy: Psychological treatments of co-existing marital and phobic-obsessive problems. *Behaviour Analysis and Modification, 4*, 3-16.

Cobb, J., Mathews, A., Childs-Clarke, A., & Blowers, C. (1984). The spouse as co-therapist in the treatment of agoraphobia. *British Journal of Psychiatry, 44*, 282-287.

Emmelkamp, P. M. G. (1974). Self-observation versus flooding in the treatment of agoraphobia. *Behaviour Research and Therapy, 12*, 229-237.

Emmelkamp, P. M. G. (1980). Agoraphobics' interpersonal problems. *Archives of General Psychiatry, 37*, 1303-1306.

Emmelkamp, P. M. G. (1982). In vivo treatment of agoraphobia. in D. L. Chambless & A. J. Goldstein (Eds.), *Agoraphobia*. New York: Wiley.

Emmelkamp, P. M. G., & Mersch, P. P. (1982). Cognition and exposure in vivo in the treatment of agoraphobia: Short-term and delayed effects. *Cognitive Research and Therapy, 6*, 77-90.

Emmelkamp, P. M. G., & Van der Hout, A. (1982). Failure in treating agoraphobia. In E. B. Foa & P. M. G. Emmelkamp (Eds.), *Failures in behavior therapy*. New York: John Wiley.

Falloon, I. R. H., Boyd, J. L., & McGill, C. W. (1984). *Family care of schizophrenia*. New York: Guilford Press.

Fisch, R., Weakland, J. H., & Segal, L. (1982). *The tactics of change*. San Francisco: Jossey-Bass.

Fodor, I. E. (1974). The phobic syndrome in women. In V. Franks & V. Burtle (Eds.), *Women in therapy*. New York: Brunner/Mazel.

Freud, S. (1932). *New introductory lectures on psychoanalysis*. London: Hogarth Press.

Fry, W. (1962). The marital context of an anxiety syndrome. *Family Process, 1*, 245-252.

Goldstein, A. J. (1982). Agoraphobia: Treatment successes, treatment failures, and theoretical implications. In D. L. Chambless & A. J. Goldstein (Eds.), *Agoraphobia*. New York: Wiley.

Goldstein, A. J. & Chambless, D. L. (1978). A reanalysis of agoraphobia. *Behavior Therapy, 9*, 47-59.

Goodstein, R., & Swift, K. (1977). Psychotherapy with phobic patients: The marriage relationship as the source of symptoms and the focus of treatment. *American Journal of Psychotherapy, 31*, 285-292.

Guidano, V. F., & Liotti, G. (1983). *Cognitive processes and emotional disorders*. New York: Guilford Press.

Hafner, R. J. (1976). Fresh symptom emergence after intensive behaviour therapy. *British Journal of Psychiatry, 129*, 378-383.

Hafner, R. J. (1977). The husbands of agoraphobic women: Assortative mating or pathogenic interaction? *British Journal of Psychiatry, 130*, 233-239.

Hafner, R. J. (1981). Spouse-aided therapy in psychiatry: An introduction. *Australian and New Zealand Journal of Psychiatry, 15*, 329-337.

Hafner, R. J. (1982). The marital context of the agoraphobic syndrome. In D. L. Chambless & A. J. Goldstein (Eds.), *Agoraphobia*. New York: Guilford.

Hafner, R. J. (1984). The marital repercussions of behavior therapy for agoraphobia. *Psychotherapy, 4*, 530-542.

Haley, J. (1976). *Problem-solving therapy*. San Francisco: Jossey-Bass.

Haley, J. (1980). *Leaving home*. New York: McGraw-Hill.

Hand, I., & Lamontagne, Y. (1976). The exacerbation of inter-personal problems after rapid phobia removal. *Psychotherapy: Theory, research & practice*, 1976, *13*, 405-411.

Hand, I., Spochring, B., & Stanik, E. (1977). Treatment of obsessions, compulsions and phobias as hidden couple-counseling. In J. C. Boulogouris & A. D. Rabavilas (Eds.), *The treatment of phobic and obsessive-compulsive disorders*. Oxford: Pergamon Press, 1977.

Hoffman, L. (1981). *Foundations of family therapy*. New York: Basic Books.

Hoover, C. F., & Insel, T. R. (1984). Families of origin in obsessive-compulsive disorder. *Journal of Nervous and Mental Diseases, 172*, 207-215.

Jacobs, R., Miller, M., Turner, S., & Wall, C. (1985). Otoneurological examination in panic disorder and agoraphobia with panic attacks: A pilot study. *American Journal of Psychiatry, 142*, 715-720.

Kuhn, T. (1962). *The structure of scientific revolutions*. University of Chicago Press.

Lazarus, A. (1966). Broad-spectrum behavior therapy and the treatment of agoraphobia. *Behaviour Research and Therapy, 4*, 95-97.

Liebowitz, M. R., & Klein, D. F. (1982). Agoraphobia: Clinical features, pathophysiology, and treatment. In D. L. Chambless & A. J. Goldstein (Eds.), *Agoraphobia*. New York: Wiley.

Liotti, G., & Guidano, V. (1976). Behavioural analysis of marital interaction in agoraphobic male patients. *Behaviour Research and Therapy, 14*, 161-162.

Madanes, C. (1981). *Strategic family therapy*. San Francisco: Jossey-Bass.

Marks, I. M. (1981). New developments in psychological treatments of phobias. In M. Mavissikalian & D. H. Barlow (Eds.), *Phobia*. New York: Guilford Press.

Marks, I. M., & Herst, E. R. (1970). A survey of 1200 agoraphobics in Britain. *Social Psychiatry, 5*, 16-24.

Mathews, A., Teasdale, J., Munby, M., Johnston, J. D., & Shaw, P. (1977). A home-based treatment program for agoraphobia. *Behavior Therapy, 8*, 915-924.

Mathews, A. M., Gelder, M. G., & Johnston, D. W. (1981). *Agoraphobia: Nature and treatment*. New York: Guilford Press.

Michelson, L., & Mavissikalian, M. (1985). Psychophysiological outcome of behavioral and pharmacological treatments of agoraphobia. *Journal of Consulting and Clinical Psychology, 53*, 229-236.

Milton, F., & Hafner, R. J. (1979). The outcome of behavior therapy for agoraphobia in relation to marital adjustment. *Archives of General Psychiatry, 36*, 807-811.

Minuchin, S. (1974). *Families and family therapy*. Cambridge, MA: Harvard University Press.

Quadrio, C. (1983). Rapunzel and the pumpkin-eater: Marital systems of agoraphobic women. *Australian Journal of Family Therapy, 4*, 81-85.

Rohrbaugh, M., & Eron, J. B. (1982). The strategic systems therapies. In L. E. Abt & I. R. Stuart (eds.), *The newer therapies: A sourcebook*. New York: Van Nostrand Reinhold.

Rosenhan, F. L. & Seligman, M. E. P. (1984). *Abnormal psychology*. New York: W.W. Norton.

Selvini Palazzoli, M., Boscolo, L., Cecchin, G., & Prata, G. (1978). *Paradox and counterparadox*. New York: Jason Aronson.

Sheehan, D. V. (1982). Panic attacks and phobias. *New England Journal of Medicine, 307*, 156-158.

Sheehan, D. V. (1983). *The anxiety disease*. New York: Scribner's.

Solyom, L., Silberfeld, M., & Solyom, C. (1976). Maternal overprotection in the etiology of agoraphobia. *Canadian Psychiatric Association Journal, 21*, 109-113.

Telch, M. J., Tearnan, B. H., & Taylor, C. B. (1983). Antidepressant medication in the treatment of agoraphobia: A critical review. *Behaviour Research and Therapy, 21*, 505-517.

Thyer, B., Neese, R., Cameron, O., & Curtis, G. (1985). Agoraphobia: A test of the separation anxiety hypothesis. *Behavior Research and Therapy, 23*, 75-78.

Tucker, D. W. (1956). Diagnosis and treatment of the phobic reaction. *American Journal of Psychiatry, 112*, 825-830.

Tyrer, P., Candy, J., & Kelly, D. (1973). A study of the clinical effects of phenelzine and placebo in the treatment of phobic anxiety. *Psychopharmacologia, 32*, 237-254.

Vandereycken, W. (1983). Agoraphobia and marital relationship: Theory, treatment and research. *Clinical Psychology Review, 3*, 317-336.

Watzlawick, P., & Weakland, J. H. (1977). *The international view*. New York: W.W. Norton.

Watzlawick, P., Weakland, J. H., & Fisch, R. (1974). *Change*. New York: W.W. Norton.

Weakland, J. H., Fisch, R., Watzlawick, P., & Bodin, A. (1974). Brief therapy: Focused problem resolution. *Family Process, 13*, 141-168.

Webster, A. S. (1953). The development of phobias in married women. *Psychological Monographs, 67* (Whole No. 367).

Westphal, C. (1871-72). Die agoraphobie: Eine neuropathische erschein. *Archiv für Psychiatrie und Nervenkrankheiten, 3*, 138-171, 219-221.

Families
and Eating Disorders

Richard Schwartz

The field of eating disorders and the field of family therapy arose from different theoretical traditions and developed independently of each other until the early 1970s. At that time the two fields intersected in a brief and tumultuous encounter. Since then, they have maintained a relationship characterized by mutual suspicion mixed with curiosity. This chapter will sketch the history of this relationship between the two fields and then will explore its legacy for the practitioner who is not wedded to either. Thus, I hope to capture some of the advances in the conceptualization and treatment of anorexia nervosa, and her younger sibling bulimia, that accrued after therapists and researchers began to look outside as well as inside their patients for clues.

BACKGROUND

Until the early 1960s bulimia was relatively unknown and anorexia nervosa was viewed in the field of eating disorders primarily as either a psychophysiological reaction involving an endocrine imbalance or, from the analytic tradition, as a fear of sex or impregnation. Through the lens provided by either of these perspectives, investigators could see only the internal workings of the patient because their vision blurred when examining aspects of her[1] context, whether that context was familial or sociocultural. Indeed, to the psychophysiologists, family or other environmental factors were largely irrelevant. To the analysts the family, when it was considered, was commonly viewed as a

Reprint requests may be addressed to Richard Schwartz, Family Systems Program, Institute for Juvenile Research, 907 South Wolcott, Chicago, IL 60612.

noxious influence which the therapist was impotent to change and from which the patient should be protected or removed.

Autonomy and Early Development

In the early 1960s the goosechase for the one physiological flaw or sexual symbol behind anorexia nervosa was slowed dramatically by a new perspective. Hilde Bruch tied anorexic symptoms to the patient's struggle for autonomy and identity within the family context that stifled these qualities (Bruch, 1963, 1973). She hypothesized that an anorexic's lack of differentiation from her mother early in the anorexic's life left her unable to identify hunger correctly. Thus Bruch added the patient's interpersonal context, largely her past interactions with her mother, to the formula for anorexia nervosa. This contribution, while incomplete, particularly in its emphasis on past causes and on blaming the patient's mother, did lift the exploration out of an interpersonal morass and paved the way for advances to come.

Indeed, statements in Bruch's later writing foreshadowed these advances. In addressing the prognosis of anorexia, she writes, "In my experience this favorable course depends to an extent on the way families become involved in the treatment process" (Bruch, 1973, p. 85). Thus she clearly recognized the importance of the anorexic's family context and the therapist's responsibility to work with it.

Thus we see several different perspectives regarding the relationship between the family and anorexia nervosa emerging from the field of eating disorders. The family was seen by some as (1) irrelevant, by others as (2) an unalterable noxious influence on the patient-as-victim, and by still others as (3) a changeable noxious influence to be reckoned with. These remain the three dominant views of the family — in reverse order of popularity — within the field of eating disorders. Each perspective is "linear" in the sense that a sick family is seen as the cause of the problem in perspective (2) and (3) whereas biochemistry is the cause in (1). Each perspective also results in very different approaches to the family in treatment. The family will be ignored by those who hold the first perspective. Those who hold the second view will encourage the patient to learn to cope with rather than change their difficult family, or they will attempt a "parentectomy" through long-term residential treatment. The third view lends itself to a mode of family therapy in which the destructive behaviors of family members are pointed out to them by the therapist and patient.

Protective Function of Symptom

Bruch also devoted some attention to the sociocultural aspects of eating disorders, a level of observation that is even farther from the strictly internal focus than the family perspective. For example, she states that,

> Whatever its purpose and meaning, food refusal would be an ineffective tool in a setting of poverty and food scarcity. To all anorexic patients with whom I am familiar, even to those of lower economic background, food was available in abundance and its refusal had an enormously disorganizing effect on their families. (Bruch, 1973, p. 13)

This statement contains the seeds of a shift in thinking about the meaning of this symptom in addition to the expanded focus. Here Bruch hints that food refusal might be a tool, might have a function or play a role within the family rather than simply be the product of disturbed family interactions. She did not pursue this perspective of symptoms however, from which eating problems are viewed as not only influenced by but also influencing (often protecting) their context.

Independent of the family therapy field, a group of prominent eating disorder experts began to speculate about the protective nature of anorexia nervosa in families based on a study of the reaction of parents to improvements in their child's symptoms (Crisp, Harding & McGuiness, 1974). They found that as the patients gained weight, most parents in their sample became more "psychoneurotically disturbed" rather than less. They conclude that "the daughter's illness sometimes serves a protective function for one or both parents as well as the patient, especially if the marital relationship is poor and acutely threatened by the prospect of their child's independence" (p. 172).

While new to those in the eating disorders field, ideas regarding the protective interplay between a symptomatic child and his or her family were commonplace among "systems-oriented" family therapists. The systemic thinking of family therapy was introduced to the field of eating disorders very dramatically in the pages of *Self Starvation*, a book by Mara Selvini Palazzoli (1974) who was a prominent theorist on eating disorders from the analytic tradition. Palazzoli began writing this book on anorexia from her analytic perspective so most of the book is on the intrapsychic life of the patients. In the later chapters, however, Palazzoli describes her growing frustration with the constraints of that model and with the ineffective individual treatment it spawned. After exposure to the ideas of Gregory Bateson and other

systems writers in the late 1960s, Selvini totally reorganized her thinking about the relationship between anorexia nervosa and its context,
and also reorganized her treatment approach. This shift in conceptual
models produced a remarkable change in both the content and the
tenor of her writing. It is as if the first two-thirds and the last third of
the book were written by different people. Compare the following
statements about the context of anorexia, the first taken from page 109
and the second from page 232: "... the therapist's dealings with the
parents should be confined to occasional suggestions on how they
should behave towards the patient and to fostering optimism and faith
in the outcome even during the worst crises," versus, "I am referring
explicitly to the common error of Western thought (and hence of psychiatry) — the idea that there is a self capable of transcending the system."

Selvini's new appreciation of the importance of the anorexic's family system and the role the patient played in protecting it from changes
the family might perceive as dangerous, inspired her and her colleagues to develop a powerful and influential model of therapy known
as the Milan Model (Selvini Palazzoli et al., 1978).

The therapist who uses the Milan Model meets with the family in
monthly sessions and inquires, from a neutral position, about the relationships among the family members, often including several generations. Once enough information has been gathered for the therapist (or
therapy team, since therapy is commonly practiced with an observing
team behind a mirror) to form an hypothesis regarding the evolution of
the current network of family relationships in which the anorexic
symptoms are embedded, that hypothesis is relayed to the family in
the form of a "positive connotation" intervention in which the patient
is restrained from giving up her symptomatic behavior for fear of up-
setting the delicate balance of family relationships that it protects. In
this way the patient's behavior is reframed as sacrificial and altruistic
rather than as selfish, rebellious, or crazy, and the family's "game" is
exposed. The Milan group reports that such positive connotations often provoke sudden shifts in family relationships such that the symptoms are no longer necessary.

The Milan Model, with its one session per month format, its total
deemphasis of individual in favor of family dynamics and its claims of
sudden and dramatic cures, is about as far a departure as is possible
from traditional psychoanalytic beliefs and practices. It may be that
after seeing the strange things that exposure to systemic thought did to
Palazzoli, the rest of the eating disorder field decided to avoid such
potent ideas for fear of a similar fate. For whatever reason, I am aware

of no prominent writers from the eating disorders field who have followed Palazzoli into the world of family systems theory.

Flawed Family Structure

There were those, however, who crossed the boundary between the two fields from the other direction. Salvador Minuchin and his colleagues in Philadelphia burst into the field of eating disorders armed with an outcome study reporting results never before achieved with anorexia nervosa, and with a well-developed model of family functioning and treatment called structural family therapy (Minuchin, Rosman & Baker, 1978). This outcome study had a potent impact on both the fields of family therapy and of eating disorders. These results were hailed as the first clear evidence of what family therapists had been claiming for years; that family therapy was more effective than intrapsychic individual therapy (the most common approach to anorexia).

In the field of eating disorders, the results were attacked by some, ignored by others and celebrated by a few. This initial reaction was predictable for several reasons. First, Minuchin was like the proverbial new kid on the block, who not only moved in but also challenged all the ideas of the neighborhood leaders. This challenge was returned in the form of a wide variety of criticisms about the data. The onslaught of criticism from Sours (1980), Swift (1982), Tseng and McDermott (1979) and Malone (1979) ranged from the fact that some of the patients requested individual therapy after the family stabilized, to the short follow-up (2-2/3 year average), to the lack of data on menses. While many of these shortcomings were valid, they are shared by many previous outcome studies on anorexia nervosa that were not similarly attacked. Thus this extraordinary reaction can be interpreted as more than an attempt to maintain academic standards; it represents the response of one paradigm (individually-oriented) to perturbation by another (systems-oriented family).

Despite this challenging response, the Minuchin group's results had an undeniable impact on the treatment of anorexia nervosa. Treatment centers that do not incorporate some involvement of the patient's family members are difficult to find these days. Therapists all over the country were inspired or challenged to take on "enmeshed" families *mano-a-mano*. It has been my experience, however, that relatively few of these therapists were inspired to get training in structural or any other type of family therapy before they struggled with anorexic families. These clinicians often carry their old frame of patient-as-victim-of-noxious-family into family sessions. The unfortunate result is often that the therapist and patient team up to browbeat her guilt-ridden parents to a tortuous degree. Or, on the other extreme, parents are prodded to oppressively control their rebellious food-refuser by therapists who have viewed the dramatic videotapes of Minuchin pushing parents to force their critically emaciated child to eat and assume that structural family therapy generally involves such extreme measures.

Contrary to both extremes, the structural family therapist attempts to identify and activate the strengths of an enmeshed anorexic family such that each family member gains a greater sense of autonomy and wider range of alternative behaviors. The structural view maintains that an anorexic's context, of which the family is the most significant part, will limit and shape her identity. Certain aspects of her personality or orientation to life will be overdeveloped and other "partial selves" will be underdeveloped (Minuchin, et al., 1978). This view implies that a family context can be restructured, that is, the obstacles to competent functioning cleared away, such that underdeveloped partial selves are activated and nurtured in all family members.

Anorexia is seen as an attempt to distract the family made necessary by the inability of the family to resolve conflicts or navigate through developmental changes. The therapist gets close enough to family members to use his or her relationship as a lever for promoting the direct negotiating of avoided conflicts, often involving the defining of more appropriate boundaries between family members.

Comparing Family Models

To briefly compare structural family therapy with the Milan Model, the other form of family therapy influential with eating disorders, both models share a view of the family as a cybernetic organism or organization, one that constantly regulates its own functioning. One major conceptual difference between the structural perspective and that of the Milan group is in the way each views the fit between the symptom and the family. Where Palazzoli emphasized the meaning or protective function that anorexia held within the complex web of family relationships, Minuchin et al. were more interested in the organizational flaw, the dysfunction in the family's structure, that maintains the anorexia. To provide a very oversimplified example of this difference, Palazzoli might focus on the resourceful way that Mary, the patient, has found to keep her mother occupied, by not eating so that mother will not bother father who is still attached to his mother, and so on. Minuchin, with the same family, might, at least initially, concentrate on the way that the parents interfere with each other when they try to get Mary to eat, with the goal of getting them to work together so that Mary is no longer the battleground for their issues.

This and other seemingly minor differences in conceptualizing problems result in extremely different sets of therapy behaviors between the structural and Milan approaches. Thus, even when coming from the same conceptual tradition, slightly different ideas about the relationship between a problem and its context are magnified enormously when they are translated into practice. This phenomenon highlights the importance of continually examining one's ideas concerning this relationship between eating problems and context relative to those presented in this paper.

Bulimia

Thus, the family context of anorexia nervosa has been systematically charted and family therapy is an increasingly accepted part of treatment for that symptom. One would expect that in light of the apparent advances made in the understanding and treatment of anorexia nervosa after the family context of the problem was examined more fully, the families of bulimics would have been carefully scrutinized by now. To the best of my knowledge, this is not the case. It is rare to find descriptions of bulimic families that rely on more than reports of patients. This absence of consideration of family context in the literature on bulimia may be partially explained by the high average age of most samples of bulimics, relative to anorexic samples. That is, because they are older, many bulimics are no longer living with their families of origin; therapists are thus less likely to include the families in treatment. In addition, many bulimics try to be secretive about their symptoms, and may claim that their families do not know about the bulimia and hence should not be involved. This attitude is epitomized by a recent unsupported statement about treating bulimia by Donald Keppner (in Cunningham, 1984):

> Most of the time family therapy is totally out of the question . . . the family would totally, utterly refuse to come into treatment. . . . Changing the system you're in isn't a real good philosophy. I think we should learn to cope with the people in our environment and not hope they will change.

Needless to say, I disagree. I have also found that while it is often true that a bulimic believes her family does not know about the bulimia, it is rare to find that family members do not have some awareness of it, and even more rare that they are unwilling to participate. In addition, I have treated many bulimics who live away from home, and have found that despite their geographical separation, they are still quite involved with their families. Thus, I believe that it is just as important to understand bulimia in the family context as it is to do so for anorexia nervosa.

EATING DISORDERS IN CONTEXT

My colleagues and I have attempted to fill this gap in the understanding of bulimia by systematically comparing our experiences with the hundreds of bulimic patients and their families that we treated over the past six years (Schwartz, Barrett & Saba, 1985). In addition, we intensively studied the characteristics of a sample of 30 bulimic patients and their families. Below I will describe some of our findings and present an hypothesis to explain the similarities that eating disordered families share.

Minuchin et al., (1978) described five interaction patterns that they believe characterize anorexic families, as well as other psychosomatic families. These include enmeshment, over-protectiveness, rigidity, lack of conflict resolution, and involvement of the patient in parental conflict. These five characteristics have been quite apparent in nearly all of the bulimic families we have studied, and to this list we would add three more: isolation, consciousness of appearances, and a special meaning attached to food and eating. In studying our sample we began to notice that, while all these characteristics were evident in all the families, the issues that these characteristics revolved around differed depending on the family's cultural history or context.

Once we began to examine the larger context and the heritage of the families, their dysfunctional characteristics, mentioned above, began to make more sense. That is, we noticed that while all the families seemed, for example, enmeshed, hyperconscious of appearances, or overprotective, the issues around which these characteristics have been played out largely depended on the degree to which the family is "Americanized" (i.e., striving to achieve the dominant values of our culture) is "ethnic" (holding the values of their culture-of-origin) or is in-between (i.e., holding some ethnic and some American values). Among our sample of 30 families, about one-third (33%) were clearly "ethnic" families; about 40% showed a blend of ethnic and American values ("mixed" families); and about 27% were predominantly "all-American" families. Rather than viewing these three classes of families, the ethnic, mixed, and all-American, as discrete categories, I see them as ranges of variation on a continuum of the degree of evolution of family values and structure. To briefly illustrate one of the differences among the three types of families, I will describe the different messages each family might give the patient about her weight or eating. In all-American families there is a strong value on competing to appear stylish (which in the United States means to be thin) at all times. The comical television phrase that "it is better to look good than to feel good" is a credo of these families. Particularly for the women in these families, esteem and parental approval hangs on one's weight.

In contrast, ethnic families, while also containing strong pressure to appear a certain way, i.e., to maintain traditional roles, showed far less aversion to fitness; indeed, it was common to find several obese family members. A mother's competence was often defined by how well or much her family ate, and a father's by how well he "brought home the bacon." In these families food and what one did with it became a central arena for defining relationships — for expressing love or anger — whereas in the all-American families relationships were defined by who looked best — was thinnest.

In the third group of "mixed" families the patient felt the pull of contradictory ethnic and American values. Around food this was manifested by both the eat-or-you-don't-love-me message coupled with the don't-be-a-pig/don't-get-fat injunction. Thus the conflicting ethnic and American messages make for a confused relationship with food. These and other differences among the three groups of families suggested an hypothesis regarding the evolution of the dysfunctional family characteristics that I have found useful both in understanding and in developing goals for the treatment of eating disordered, as well as other types of families.

Cultural/Evolutionary Hypothesis

Why are the families of bulimics or anorexics so enmeshed, overprotective, appearance-conscious, triangulating (e.g., involving children in the parent's marriage), rigid, and so forth? Why are the parents so nonassertive, dependent, afraid to grow up? Is it because of deepseated intrapsychic pathology that permeates the character of key family members? Family therapists would like to think not, but we have few useful alternative explanations.

If a family's lineage is traced far enough, one will usually find that at one point or another in its history, the family was embedded within a stable kin network. The families within many such networks will have many characteristics that are functional and adaptive for existence in that context but are not so adaptive outside the network. For example, there is little need for, nor is it easy to have, a close, intimate relationship between the parents of a family surrounded by close relatives. The father has his network of male friends, the mother spends time with her mother and sisters, and everybody is involved in everybody else's conflicts. The children will not leave the network after they become adults, so there is little need for parents to support each other in preparation for an empty nest. Network loyalty is paramount; as a result of historical invasions by or conflicts with other groups, the extra-familial is feared. Children are raised to be obedient and loyal rather than personally ambitious. Finally, food is a central focus of interaction and ritual within the network.

The family structure and values described above, which are fully adaptive for a stable network, may create problems if the family leaves the network and becomes a part of bountiful, mobile middle America, unless the family's structure can change rapidly. The family is likely to maintain its distrust of strangers, and consequently to become extremely isolated. The parents, not knowing how to get close to each other or not being oriented to do so, are likely to become over-involved with their children and to discourage them from leaving. From their family, the children will get large doses of the loyalty ethic and yet will feel the pull of values for personal success and independence that permeate their environment outside the family family. After some time, the parents may give the patient contradictory push-pull messages as one or both of them become imbued with ambition, yet their family structure may not have restructured enough to permit fulfillment of these ambitions, i.e., to allow the autonomy and mobility necessary for the ambitious child.

This isolation, lack of marital closeness, and child-centeredness leads family members to "feed off" one another. They become so interdependent that the family is hypersensitive to any threat to the marriage or to the demeanor of the parents or to the possible departure of key members. In short, all family members come to believe that the cohesion of the family is quite delicate, and they organize to avoid change. After several generations adrift in the American mainstream, values of competitiveness and vogue appearance may prevail in the family, but the basic structure may still be retained from the network.

The following interchange illustrates the predicament of an "ethnic" family that has not adapted; in this case, a withdrawn 22-year-old bulimic and her first-generation Italian parents.

Consultant:	(*To mother*) Sally (the patient) says she is very worried about you and about your husband. She thinks you wouldn't make it if she grew up.
Sally:	(*Weakly*) That's right.
Mother:	That's crazy. Why should she worry about our relationship? Nobody's happy all the time.
Consultant:	I don't think she worries about you two splitting up; I don't think there's much chance of that. I think she thinks you will be sad. You have been a mother a long time. You have four kids? How old is the youngest?
Mother:	Eighteen.
Consultant:	Sally seems to worry that soon they will be gone, and then what will you do?
Mother:	That's crazy. I don't want her worrying about me — she has her own problems. I never worried about my mother. She had ten kids and they never worried about her.
Consultant:	Was your mother's mother around then? And her sisters and friends?
Mother:	Yes.
Consultant:	Then no wonder you didn't have to worry about her. Is your mother around?
Mother:	No.
Consultant:	Any sisters or brothers around?
Mother:	No, they are still in Italy.
Consultant:	Do you have many friends?
Mother:	I see what you're getting at, but I don't want her worrying about me. She has her own life to think of.

This model of evolution of enmeshed families and their associated problems is not intended to apply to all families with eating disorders. Instead, it is presented as an over-arching framework that implies that if the therapist is able to help the family or individual change or better accommodate to their context, then the problems will abate. In some cases, this may mean getting the parents to support each other; in other cases, it may mean helping them open their boundaries to establish a new network. In yet others, it may be possible to help the patient establish a network for herself apart from the family without having to involve other family members directly. In general, however, this model implies a view of eating disorder symptoms as an adaptive solution for a family whose structure has not fully adapted to its context.

Why are women so much more vulnerable to eating disorders than men? In addition to the omnipresent pressure on women in American society to look unhealthily thin, eating disordered families tend to give their children conflicting messages about their roles.

Patients who are raised amid these delicate, interdependent, stuck families tend to develop extreme "partial selves" or internal pasts that reflect the conflicting values of their family. That is, a part of many patients is oriented toward achieving a lot—living up to her great potential—and becomes perfectionistically critical when she is not constantly working toward that goal. Another internal part is oriented toward being perfectly "feminine" in the traditional or ethnic sense, i.e., toward sacrificing for others (particularly men), doing domestic things and staying home. This "domestic" part is likely to believe that she does not deserve nor should she ask for much in life. The conflicts generated from these internal parts and by messages from family and society, may leave these young women confused, feeling incompetent and in need of a distraction or way to avoid moving in either direction. The patients' obsession with food or weight provides such a method of avoiding these contextual and life cycle issues for both her and for her family.

TREATMENT

The model of therapy my colleagues and I have developed is designed to help families restructure so as to provide a better fit with their context, and, relatedly, help the patient restructure her internal extremes. In so doing we have primarily drawn from the structural and the strategic schools of family therapy. Structural family therapy (Minuchin, 1974; Minuchin & Fishman, 1981; Minuchin et al., 1978) has been unfairly stereotyped by many practitioners in the field of eating disorders who have seen or heard about a few dramatic videotapes ("Structuralists? Oh yeah, they're the people who force anorexics to eat hot dogs!"). What such stereotypes miss in that assessment is a way of viewing people that is extremely optimistic and allows the therapist to scan for and elicit the strengths rather than the deficits in people. The idea is that an individual's context, of which the family is a very significant part, will limit and shape a person's experience in such a way that certain "partial selves" (i.e., aspects of their personality and orientation to life) will be overaccessed by them and other "partial selves" underaccessed.

As applied to eating symptoms, this model suggests that in spite of appearing to be hopelessly nonassertive, self-deprecating, or enmeshed with her family, the patient has the ability to behave and think in very different, more competent ways. Thus, large doses of education, insight, behavior modification, or medication need not be doled out by the therapist, because it is assumed that the individual and family already have within them the ability to be competent, and will do so if released from habitual interaction patterns and orientations that have fostered the fear of change.

This model of change translates into a directive style of therapy where, in family sessions, family members are encouraged and challenged to interact in new ways and to see themselves and one another differently. Relationships that have been blocked or interfered with in the past are reengaged and strengthened. The reinforcing aspect of this process is that family members get to know and affirm one another beyond the masks (partial selves) they habitually show one another. This is an extremely important part of working with eating disordered families, because the family members tend to have very rigid images of themselves and one another.

In addition to the structural orientations described above, I have also been conceptually and technically influenced by strategic and systemic family therapies and their concern with and respect for (1) the ambivalence that families and individuals have regarding change; (2) the consequences of change; (3) the importance of the sequences of interactions and thinking that surround the symptom (Fisch, Weakland, & Segal, 1982; Haley, 1976; Madanes, 1981; Selvini Palazzoli, Boscolo, Cecchin, & Prata, 1978). As my colleagues and I worked with bulimic families, these considerations became increasingly salient as we recognized the degree of fear that many patients had about giving up their symptoms and the fears that many of the families had about their daughters growing up.

The techniques of strategic family therapists reflect both a concern about using or not provoking the family's or individual's resistance to change, and their search for interactional solutions to specific problems. Regarding the first concern, families or individuals are sometimes restrained by the therapist from changing too fast. They may be asked to devote a great deal of thought to the possible negative consequences of symptom remission or of various structural modifications. As the therapist promotes this protective restraining position, the family members and/or the patient often open up enough to explore the validity of their fears and inclinations to protect one another, and the side of their ambivalence that wants change often enters the foreground.

Structural/Strategic

Combining the complementary aspects of structural and strategic family therapy conceptual frameworks and techniques has not been a smooth process and is not recommended to the inexperienced family therapist. The style of therapy that has evolved from this process is one in which the therapist's position will alternate between advocating changes and warning against the same changes, in rhythm with the oscillation of the ambivalence of the family or patient. The degree of restraining necessary has varied considerably from case to case, but having that position as an alternative provides the therapist with a great deal of flexibility, so that he or she can avoid being inducted into power struggles centering on change.

The successful implementation of this rhythmic restraining—encouraging stance requires some reorienting of the therapist's attitude toward change. If the therapist views the symptom as a family's and/or an individual's response to their particular contextual predicament, rather than as a problem to be eradicated as quickly as possible, it will be easier for the therapist to focus on and nurture changes in the "big picture" (i.e., patterns of interaction and orientation), rather than becoming attached to the waxing and waning of the symptom itself. The therapist will be able to restrain with sincerity, rather than as an attempt to trick the family, because the therapist, along with the family, is aware of and respectful of the dangers in overly abrupt change. To adopt such an attitude, it is important for the therapist to understand the symptom at many levels simultaneously—that is, to view it in its full context, which may include the cultural evolutionary considerations mentioned earlier as well as specific family or individual interaction patterns.

The level of understanding advocated above is not essential to the successful treatment of some cases of bulimia, or anorexia nervosa. This is because, from case to case, there is a wide range in the level or degree of involvement of various systems in the problem. Thus, some cases can be lastingly improved with approaches that are not particularly context-sensitive. My colleagues and I are convinced, however, that in many cases we have encountered, the symptoms would not have improved or would have improved only temporarily if the patients had been treated without awareness of their context.

Internal Process

There have been occasions, particularly in working with bulimics, where the patient's family had restructured to the point where, theoretically, her symptoms should remit, and yet they did not. There seemed to be sequences of internal process within the patient's mind that had a momentum of their own, unaltered by the changes in her family, that were maintaining the symptoms. Several years ago I decided that to adequately treat such cases I needed a model of internal process that was congruent with a systemic orientation toward families. The existing models of internal process of which I was aware were incompatible with my systems viewpoint so I was forced to formulate my own framework from my patients' descriptions of what happened inside of them. They typically described the interactions of an array of parts or subpersonalities that fight with each other and take control of the person at one time or another. What was most remarkable was the similarity across patients of the types of parts they described and the sequences of the interaction among the parts that led to a binge or fast. Also remarkable was the degree to which the qualities and patterns of these internal parts matched the values and extreme interaction patterns of the patients' families, which were described earlier in this chapter.

A typical internal sequence leading to a food binge will involve three or four of these parts. For example, the patient may perceive that someone has slighted or criticized her. This perception will activate a part of her that is extremely critical of her in many areas—her personality, her level of achievement and, of course, her looks. (This part often tells her not to eat at all because she is such a pig.) In turn, a part that defends her against this critical part will be activated and she may lash out against the person who provoked the sequence. Also aroused by the critical part, however, is a part that feels very young, helpless, sad and uncared for. These feelings are very distressing for these patients and, almost automatically, another part rescues them by taking over and making them eat. Indeed, most bulimics describe their binge episodes as dissociative experiences in which they are hardly aware of what they are doing, as if they had become unfeeling eating machines. After the binge the critical part attacks her for overeating and the sequence is repeated indefinitely.

The internal sequence I have noticed in restricter anorexics is different from that of bulimics, in that in anorexics the critical, perfectionistic part is more dominant in the internal system and joins forces with a part that protects the patient by telling her to withdraw, and to override the other parts. Thus with anorexics one does not find the mood swings that are characteristic of bulimics and, instead, the therapist continually faces this coalition of parts that take over and distort the anorexic's perceptions, from what people say to her to what she sees in the mirror. Thus, other parts exist within her but are stifled by this "dictatorship."

These differences in internal sequences between anorexics and bulimics are consistent with observations of the characteristics of their respective families. That is, bulimic families are generally more labile and conflictual than anorexic families, in which "self-control" and striving for perfection are more notable.

I have designed a model for understanding and intervening into these systems of internal parts (Schwartz, 1987) that is consistent with and isomorphic to the structural/strategic model I hold for families. With this framework I can now move fluidly between the internal and family levels of system when working with eating disorders or other types of problems. This ability has improved my effectiveness with eating disorders a great deal.

EPILOGUE

In this paper I have reviewed the relationship between the fields of eating disorders and family therapy, and I have presented some aspects of the systems-based model I use when treating these patients and their families. Let me end by saying that my work with this population has been so fascinating and also so frustrating that I have been challenged to create and explore new models of therapy and of life. I am grateful to my patients for this opportunity and for their patience with me.

NOTE

1. Throughout this paper the author has used feminine pronouns when referring to the patient because the large majority of people who have an eating disorder are female (DSM III, 1980).

REFERENCES

Bruch, H. *Eating disorders*. London: Routledge & Kegan Paul, 1974.

Bruch, H. Psychotherapeutic problems in eating disorders. *Psychoanalytic Review*, 1963, (50), 43.

Crisp, A. H., Harding, B. & McGuinness, B. Anorexia nervosa, psychoneurotic characteristics of parents: Relationship to prognosis. *Journal of Psychosomatic Research*, 1974, *18*, 167-173.

Cunningham, S. Bulimia's cycle shames patient, tests therapists. *American Psychological Association Monitor*, 1984, *15*(1), 16-17.

Diagnostic and Statistical Manual of Mental Disorders (3rd ed.), American Psychiatric Association, 1980.

Fisch, R., Weakland, J. & Segal, L. *The tactics of change*. San Francisco: Jossey-Bass, 1982.

Haley, J. *Problem-solving therapy*. San Francisco: Jossey-Bass, 1976.

Madanes, C. *Strategic family therapy*. San Francisco: Jossey-Bass, 1981.

Malone, A. Child psychiatry and family therapy. *Journal of the American Academy of Child Psychiatry*, 1979, *18*, 4-21.

Minuchin, S. *Families and family therapy*. Cambridge, MA: Harvard University Press, 1974.

Minuchin, S. & Fishman, C. *Family therapy techniques*. Cambridge, MA: Harvard University Press, 1983.

Minuchin, S., Rosman, B. & Baker, L. *Psychosomatic families: anorexia nervosa in context*. Cambridge, MA: Harvard.

Schwartz, R. C. Our multiple selves. *Family Therapy Networker*, 1987, *11*, 25-31.

Schwartz, R. C., Barrett, M. J. & Saba, G. Family therapy for bulimia. In P. Garner & P. Garfinkel, (Eds.), *The handbook for the psychotherapy of anorexia nervosa and bulimia*. New York: Guilford Press, 1985.

Schwartz, R., Barrett, M. J. & Saba, G. *The treatment of bulimic individuals and their families*. New York: Guilford, In preparation.

Selvini Palazzoli, M. *Self starvation*. London: Human Context Books, 1974.

Selvini Palazzoli, M., Boscolo, L., Cecchin, G. & Prata, G. *Paradox and counter-paradox*. New York: Jason Aronson, 1978.

Sours, J. A. *Starving to death in a sea of objects: The anorexia nervosa syndrome*. New York: Jason Aronson, 1980.

Swift, W. J. The long term outcome of early onset anorexia nervosa: A critical review. *Journal of the American Academy of Child Psychiatry*, 1982, *21*, 38-46.

Tseng, W. & McDermott, J. E. Triaxial family classification. *Journal of the American Academy of Child Psychiatry*, 1979, *18*, 22-43.

Continuities and Discontinuities in the Family Treatment of Substance Abuse

John Schwartzman

INTRODUCTION

The theoretical changes which redefined substance abuse as part of a social context began in the early 1950's, and was radical enough to be described as a paradigm shift (Kuhn, 1962). This shift transformed the problem from a totally internal one, to an aspect of an interpersonal process.

Until recently, most of the study of substance abuse and the family has followed separate distinct pathways contingent on the particular drug being studied, or stage in the life-cycle. This separation is primarily an artifact of the interest of the investigators since many systems characterized by substance abuse have more than one abusing member, in more than one generation (Cotton, 1979; Hoffman & Noem, 1975), who abuse more than one substance (Kandel, Kessler & Margulies, 1978; Liebson, Bigelow & Flamer, R., 1972). These separations and the parochialisms that have resulted from their isolation, have hindered the development of theory. Theories for the treatment of alcoholism, opiate addiction and poly-drug use have all evolved independently, yet due to the trend toward poly-drug use among abusers, this is counterproductive in the development of more useful theory.

A core aspect of future theory building is a solution to the major dissonance in the field concerning the nature of addiction about which there are a number of conflicting ideas that directly influence the goals and strategies of therapy. There is implicit contradiction between the disease model of which there are a number of variations (Poole,

Reprint requests may be addressed to John Schwartzman, PhD, Faculty, Family Institute of Chicago, 900 Lincoln Street, Evanston, IL 60201.

1985), and a systems model that assumes addiction to be an aspect of a psychosocial context, especially the family.

There are two basic components of the disease concept, clearest in alcoholism but also present in theories of other drug use. This model assumes that alcoholics, (like other addicts), cannot control their drinking due to some constitutional defect elicited by the use of any alcohol, or caused by the longtime use of alcohol. The model assumes a loss of control over drinking behavior once it begins and the inevitable progression of physical and mental deterioration. The developmental pathway of alcoholism that is generally adopted is that derived from Jellinek (1960), who described the process of physical dependence and loss of control over drinking in distinct stages. This may not be a valid description, but the devastating effects of alcohol and other drug abuse on the marital and family system are undeniable. The rate of separation and divorce among alcoholics and their spouses is seven times that of the normal population (Paulino & McCrady, 1977). Children of alcoholics are overrepresented in a number of behavior and psychological problems (El-Guebly & Offord, 1977; Fox, 1962).

At a minimum, there is much evidence that contradicts a disease model, which nonetheless remains an alluring concept. For example, Room (1977) did not find the same stages of alcoholism as described by Jellinek. The status of people's drinking problems varies widely over time (Calahan & Room 1972), and there is a substantial natural remission among alcoholics and problem drinkers (Hyman, 1976; Knupfer, Calahan & Shanks, 1978).

A number of laboratory studies of alcoholics have found no loss of control in drinking (Merry, 1966; Paredes et al., 1973). Few alcoholics define loss of control as the cause for their return to abusive drinking (Ludwig, 1972). Rates of drinking can be manipulated by rewards and consequences and are quite contextually determined, at least in laboratory studies (Nathan, Goldman, Lisman & Taylor, 1972).

Jaffe (1972) notes that addiction and physical dependence cannot be used interchangeably. Pattison (1966) states that, "addiction is not purely a purely physiological mechanism, nor is the compulsion to drink" (p. 62). The above statement is partially a response to what has been termed the "pharmacological fallacy" (Adler, 1972), that still permeates the field. This is the assumption that there is a single, specific, drug effect, irrespective of context or the individual that uses it.

More inclusively, it appears that the rates of alcoholism are at least partially culturally determined. Specific alcoholic syndromes may be characteristic of specific cultures (Bales, 1946). For example, solitary addictive drinking does not occur to any great extent in small-scale, nonindustrial societies (Marshall, 1979). Drunken deportment has been shown to be learned at the cultural level, and often functions as a "time out" (MacAndrew & Edgerton 1969). All societies allow more permissable behaviors when alcohol is consumed, but what is permissible varies widely. Despite this and a great deal of other evidence, alcoholism and the other addictions are often treated as if they were a unitary problem by therapists, having inevitable outcomes, while the effects of various aspects of the context of which they are a part are ignored.

Pattison and Kaufman (1981) note the almost complete separation, only breached since the 1970s, between alcohol studies which ignored family dynamics, and family therapy which ignored alcoholism and its treatment. One of the reasons for this split is that alcoholism is one of the few mental health problems that is primarily treated by paraprofessionals (Alcohol and Drug Problem Association, 1974), often recovering alcoholics, and family therapy is performed primarily by professionals.

The evolution of family research on alcohol has gradually transformed the locus of the problem from intrapsychic conflicts to more inclusive interactional systems. This process began with descriptions of the personalities of alcoholics, to those of their spouses, and then to their interaction. Ewing and Fox (1968) were among the first to note the interactional aspects of systems involving alcohol abuse. They describe one pattern in the alcoholic marriage as a process involving a male alcoholics' dependency eliciting his wife's protective nurturing, which is contingent on his undemanding sexuality. Drewery and Rae (1969) described wives of alcoholics as confused about male sociosexual roles which they expressed in ". . . a conflictual interplay of dependence and independence needs" (p. 615). These early studies were focused on the complementarity of personality deficits, but at least suggest the process aspects rather than totally intrapsychic explanations of alcoholism (see Steinglass [1976] review of this literature). They have been severely criticized on both methodological and theoretical grounds (Kaufman, 1982). There is little evidence for an "alcoholic" personality (Syme, 1957) or a typical personality for the spouses of alcoholics (Tarter, 1976; Edwards et al., 1973). However, both seem to run in families, in that alcoholics often have an alcoholic parent, and those who marry alcoholics are often from families in which there are alcoholic members (Rimmer & Winokur, 1972).

In family therapy, alcoholism was gradually redefined as part of a process, in that the spouse's functioning was described as the result of the stress in living with an alcoholic (Jackson, 1956). This has since evolved into the concept that drinking itself might be adaptive behavior in marital interaction which, in turn, is functional in maintaining the drinking (Ward & Faillace, 1970; Becker & Miller, 1976). A number of studies have demonstrated dysfunctional communication patterns in the alcoholic marital dyad (Steinglass et al., 1971; Foy et al., 1979; Billings et al., 1979). Gorad (1971), has described how in marital conflict, the alcoholic often can only "win" by lack of control, in that his spouse cannot make him stop drinking.

A number of researchers (Orford, 1975; Paulino & McCready, 1977), believe interaction involving alcohol is unique to each couple, and that alcoholic marriages are not a unitary group (see Olson & Killoren, 1983). They believe that their functioning varies as widely as and is not different from that of nonalcoholic couples, either in contrast to "normal" couples or those with other symptoms. This debate continues, (see Steinglass, 1985; Kaufman, 1985).

Pattison and Kaufman (1981) have described a number of themes in the current literature on family systems and alcohol and their treatment. These include patterns of family functioning and alcoholism, (Steinglass et al., 1985; Pattison & Kaufman, 1981), the effects of alcohol on family functioning, the effect on children of alcoholics (Cork, 1969; Fox, 1962), families of origin (Bowen, 1974), alcoholism's transgenerational transmission (Cotton, 1979; Wolin et al., 1979, 1980). In other words, there is an increasing awareness of more inclusive systems as a crucial aspect of the problem.

Alcohol, as a part of family process, has been described as having an adaptive, homeostatic function (Davis, Berenson, Steinglass & Davis, 1974). As Pattison and Kaufmann (1981) state, "The problems of alcoholism are not just the consequences of drinking per se, but more importantly the system functions that drinking serves in the operation of the family" (p. 208).

There are a number of salient characteristics of the families of alcoholics described in the clinical literature that may help to explain how abusive drinking can be understood as an adaptive "fit" with its context. A common characteristic of the family of origin of many alcoholics is the abuse of alcohol or drugs by a parent (Ziegler-Driscoll, 1979), explained both as a genetic susceptibility (Goodwin, 1985) or as a learned response. These families are often characterized by a minimum expression of affect or express it only when a member has been drinking (Diethelm & Barr, 1962; Mardones, 1963). There have been a number of clinical reports and studies noting the changes between intoxicated and sober interaction which have described the positive changes in the "wet" system with an actively drinking alcoholic vs. those when he/she is not drinking (Davis, Berenson, Steinglass & Davis, 1974).

A number of studies (Gerard, Saegner & Wile, 1962; Kurtines, Ball & Wood, 1978; Pettinati, 1978), found a great deal of psychopathology in abstinent alcoholics. The above suggests the functionality of alcohol abuse, in that it provides systemic solutions when present, and other problems become apparent when the abuse was absent. More generally alcohol abuse has a function in terms of responsibility. As Berenson (1976) states:

> . . . alcoholic individuals and family systems are the true split personalities or oscillating systems. In the majority of cases there is a rapid swing from the over responsible nonexperience of dryness to the under-responsible intense experience, of wetness. (p. 288)

There is clinical evidence (Steinglass, 1980) that the natural history of alcohol abuse follows that of most other systems with a chronic problem. Jackson (1956) describes the stages of adjustment to the alcoholic in the family. After some period of interaction with an alcoholic member, the system readjusts itself to his increasing dysfunction so that the system becomes self-regulating with the alcoholic not fulfilling adult expectations. As a result, these families are characterized by the confused hierarchies and cross-generational coalitions (Jacob, Favorini, Meisel et al., 1978), characteristic of any system with a chronic problem. This frequently interferes with age-appropriate differentiation of the children who are often pushed or volunteer to make up parental deficits (Bowen, 1974), or act out in an analogous fashion to the parent by abusing alcohol.

There is increasing evidence for the problems of children of alcoholics (Cork, 1969; El-Guebly & Offord, 1977). One result is a difficulty in establishing intimate relationships in their own generation. Zieger-Driscoll (1979) found that almost half of the (mostly male) alcoholics in her study, whose average was 33, were still primarily involved in their family of origin father than with someone in their own generation. Often they are isolated, have only brief relationships, or those they can tolerate only with the heavy use of alcohol. They frequently have trouble functioning without the emotional and/or financial support of their parents, similar to the pseudo-autonomy which has been used to describe heroin addicts (Ganger & Shugart, 1966; Stanton, Todd et al., 1982), in that they remain primarily involved with family of origin, either because they are symptomatic, or because they are overresponsible in trying to meet inappropriate parental needs.

If their relationships result in marriage, the use of alcohol and the responses to it function to create a context similar to that described above, that often ends in divorce (Paulino & McGrady, 1977). At the same time, as stated above, individuals who marry alcoholics often grow up in families with members who are substance abusers (Wolin, Bennett & Noonan, 1979), creating a self-maintaining system through the generations.

Some of the clinical and theoretical literature on alcoholism and the family also suggests another dynamic taking place in this context, a lack of adequate constraints in terms of rules and expectations. A high percentage of alcoholics report being "spoiled" as children (Ziegler-Driscoll, 1979). A number of prospective studies have found that boys who later became abusive drinkers were undercontrolled and impulsive as children (Jones, 1968, 1971), suggesting a learned lack of control. McClelland et al., suggests that heavy drinking was a response " . . . to a strong need for power coupled with a lack of inhibition" (1972, p. 230), which would be an adaptive deutero-learned response to a context lacking constraint. These studies are overwhelmingly based on male alcoholics. Consequently one view of alcoholism or abusive drinking, at least for males, is that it has a function similar to many other problems and elicits analogous responses within a systemic family perspective. It is one adaptive response to a context characterized by a relatively unchanging culturally-inappropriate relationship with a parent (expressed positively or negatively), and a distant, nonexistent or conflictual relationship with the other, within a cultural context that has strong demands for extrafamilial autonomy, such that this relationship interferes with these demands.

These relationships develop within more inclusive sociocultural contexts with widely-varying demands and expectations in terms of drug and alcohol use, and expectations of behavior or "drunken deportment" (Mac Andrew & Edgerton, 1969), when using alcohol and drugs, which function to maintain consumption and behavior when "under the influence" within limits, or tend to amplify its use and abuse in certain contexts.

The cultural requirements and the pseudo-solution provided by alcoholism is perhaps gender-specific. Most of the studies of alcoholics have been based on male alcoholics. Women are undiagnosed or misdiagnosed more often than male alcoholics (Gomberg, 1981). It has been found that they have lower self-esteem than do male alcoholics

(Beckman, 1975), and are more likely to be depressed, (Schukit et al., 1969). Bepko believes that the relationships between the female experience, social realities, and alcoholism have barely been explored, especially the relative powerlessness of women, to which the abuse of alcohol and its accompanying guilt and depression are an appropriate response to an oppressive context. She notes that alcohol allows both sexes to experience what are defined as attributes of the other sex and "blame" it on alcohol. As she states:

> . . . it seems apparent that in many, if not all, families in which alcoholism is a factor, an inability to acknowledge or act on feelings that run counter to the traditional sex role expectations is always present to a greater or lesser degree. Further, these conflicts regarding sex role behavior cannot be separated from the pattern of over- and underresponsibility that emerge in the family. (1985, p. 56)

It is interesting to note that cross-culturally, males act out the male role in their use of alcohol in that they generally drink more and their "drunken deportment" is generally more aggressive, boisterous and dangerous than is female "drunken deportment," caricatures of their sober roles (Marshall, 1979).

One area almost completely ignored in the treatment of alcoholism, is those regulators at the cultural level which define the appropriate use of alcohol, appropriate drinking behavior and responses to inappropriate behavior which constrain it. For example, it has been suggested that the use of alcohol in rituals themselves is perhaps homeostatic in terms of limiting abuse in the groups celebrating the ritual (Marshall, 1979). In fact, people engage in socially disruptive drinking only in secular settings (Marshall, 1979).

Wolin, Bennett and their colleagues in a number of papers (Wolin, Bennett et al., 1980; Bennett & Wolin, 1984; Wolin & Bennett, 1984) have described how ritual participation is an important "comment" on family integrity in families with alcoholic members. They investigated two processes; the effects of parental alcoholism on already established family rituals, and comparisons of the children's rituals in their marital families with those of their families of origin. They found that families whose rituals were protected from disruption due to parental alcoholism resulted in less transmission of alcoholism to the next generation. In other words, the maintenance of family rituals, despite alcohol abuse, is a good prognosis for fewer problems with alcohol among the children, than those from families in which alcohol has interfered with ritual performance.

This seemed to be particularly important in terms of those individuals most at risk, sons of alcoholic fathers. Couples who did not abuse alcohol more often included spouses who were nonalcoholic and whose family had a high level of ritual performance. In their marital families, these couples maintained less contact with the alcoholic families of origin and consciously modified specific aspects of their family heritage. They found that " . . . the life course a couple chooses early in their marriage — especially in respect to heritage — is a critical consideration to their continuing or rejecting the recurrence of the alcohol problem into their own generation" (Bennett, Wolin, McAvity, n.d.; Bennet & Wolin, 1984). This suggests that the introduction of rituals might be a powerful intervention, in families characterized by substance abuse (see Schwartzman, 1983).

FAMILIES OF OPIATE ABUSERS

There are now many descriptions of the functioning of families with a member addicted to heroin (Davis & Klagsburn, 1977; Ganger & Schugart, 1968; Schwartzman, 1975, 1969; Stanton et al., 1982) from what can be termed a systemic perspective. These (again generally based on a sample of males), suggest the adaptive aspects of addiction, for the individual and the family, especially as part of a crucial homeostatic process for both in family systems that have difficulty making transitions.

The families become part of developmental dysfunction, maintaining and maintained by the opiate abuse which defocused from the often-present marital discord. At the same time, drug abuse was found to maintain the parents' relationship within tolerable limits, while permanently altering its emotional balance in the family. Often the abuser and one parent become and remain the family's most emotionally intense dyad. Disagreements between the parents about the addict maintained marital conflict and the addict's involvement in the marriage in such a way that attempts at separation and greater autonomy were undercut by family members. The result was manifest in the addict's pseudo-autonomy, leaving home failing, and being rescued again and again. This cycle was contingent on the continued chronic addiction of the addict, and on social systems that do not make culturally-appropriate transitions such as these families. Chronic addiction required only pseudo-separation by the addict. Concurrently it results in the addict's curtailed developmental cycle, since he seldom established adequate relationships with peers or later with spouses that were as intimate as was that with the family of origin. In crises, addicts often returned to their family of origin, whatever their marital status. Their success in remaining abstinent has been correlated with living away from home successfully (Vaillant, 1966).

It has been suggested that addiction itself can be seen as the ultimate sacrifice in the family, a slow suicide (Stanton, 1977). Later studies have described the many, and improperly-mourned losses that characterize these families (Coleman & Stanton, 1978). Analogous to the process suggested by Walsh (1978) in terms of many losses in families with a schizophrenic member, the surviving parent does not mourn the lost parent or spouse and instead replaces him/her with one of the children. This child is then overprotected, "helped" or seen as different in some way, especially as lacking control or judgement. When it is time for culturally-appropriate separation, there is the onset, exacerbation, or discovery of serious drug problems.

Stanton et al (1982) note many similarities of families with a member addicted to heroin with other severely dysfunctional families. At the same time, they describe a number of distinct aspects. Frequently there is alcohol abuse by a parent or other close relatives, and other out of control behavior, e.g., gambling, eating, violence, etc. It has also been hypothesized that within this context, addicts deutero-learn (Bateson, 1972) a context characterized by lack of constraint, and when behaving symptomatically, often create contexts characterized by similar processes (Schwartzman & Bokos, 1979; Schwartzman & Kroll, 1977). In addition, the addicts were characterized by more pseudo-autonomy, periods of functioning outside the family, than in other serious, chronic symptoms, perhaps as the result of an available deviant subculture. In addition, the overinvolved parents were often very isolated, (immigrants seem to be overrepresented as parents), perhaps making even more probable their overattachment to their children, in such a way as to make their culturally-appropriate separation even more difficult.

These families have problems with the communication of affect, especially anger, often either absent or inappropriately expressed. Being "high" or "under the influence" provides a pseudo-solution, in that affect can more easily be communicated and concurrently blamed on the drug.

Individuals who have utilized the abuse of alcohol and/or opiates as an adaptive mode are making a "comment" on contexts in terms of the confusions concerning the lack of responsibility for their own behavior and feelings, and their own confusions about control and lack of control. These are the issues that must be resolved in their treatment by attempting to create contexts such that this cognitive set and interpersonal style are no longer adaptive.

INTERVENTIONS

Pattison and Kaufman (1981) note the almost complete separation between alcoholism studies which ignored family dynamics and family therapy which ignored alcoholism. This dichotomy has been maintained despite alcoholism's prevalence as a symptom, an interesting isomorph to the family often characterized by massive denial in terms of its members' alcoholism.

For those families characterized by alcohol abuse primarily, there has been more emphasis on the traditional approach to alcoholism — the disease model, which assumes they are basically similar, due to the nature of alcohol. There are some clinical reports (Scott, 1970; Pattison, 1965; Meeks & Kelly, 1970), suggesting that family therapy can be effective. Pattison and Kaufman (1981) suggests an eclectic model utilizing structural strategic, psychodynamic, communication, and other approaches. Some family therapists will only work with "dry" systems, and suggest family therapy after the identified patient has stopped drinking, although it has not been demonstrated that this is the only effective approach (Pattison, 1966).

A number of family therapists assume that their job is to "confront the denial" that is, to get the patient and the family members to accept their alcoholism, with its accompanying implications, as the primary intervention in their treatment with alcoholics. Many believe that their main intervention is to get family members to go to the appropriate self-help groups, Alcoholics Anonymous, Ala-Non, Ala-teen, etc. At these meetings one of the basic interventions to family members is the prescription of psychological distance so that they not be influenced by the alcoholic's behavior in their traditional way, especially the drinking. Instead they are redefined as in charge of their own behavior and their own responses to the alcoholic. This is enacted at the level of structure because the meetings are attended separately from the alcoholic.

There are a number of descriptions for the functioning of AA (Trice, 1958; Kurtz, 1979). Its fundamental premise consists of the acceptance of the "disease" of alcoholism, and its implications, especially its permanence, lack of control over drinking, and abstinence as the only goal, in which the refusal of treatment is regarded as a manifestation of denial which suggests alcoholism. A common treatment strategy for families with an alcoholic member is to get the family to accept a relabeling of the problem as a disease, with an inevitable progression, absolving the individual and family of blame, but requiring continuing attendance at AA to maintain sobriety, and teaching this theory to other family members and the alcoholic. One of the best known family approaches, that of Berenson (1976), suggests as the initial intervention offering the alcoholic's spouse three alternatives; continue to do what she does, emotional or physical detachment, or separating or physically distancing from the alcoholic. This is congruent with Al-Anon's and other substance-abuse self-help groups' major directive of admitting powerlessness over the alcoholic's drinking, and "detaching with love," but being in control of one's own response to it. This suggests that an important theoretical task in the study of family therapy and the treatment of substance abuse, is a cybernetic understanding of the functioning of the self-help groups that are widely assumed to be the most effective form of treatment.

A work that has attempted this is Bateson's (1971) article, "The Cybernetics of Self . . . ," in which he translates the alcoholic's functioning and that of Alcoholics Anonymous, into a cybernetic perspective. He argues that the alcoholic's problem is primarily the result of Cartesian dualism in which conscious will on which the alcoholic depends for control, is separated from the unconscious forces that drive him to drink. This is manifest in alcoholic "pride" so that he must prove himself over and over to demonstrate ability to control his use of alcohol which must ultimately fail. Bateson states that alcoholics have learned only to operate in symmetrical relationships based on equality so that challenges are met in a competitive way, and will eventually fail in the context of controlled drinking. Demands that he accept his problems with controlling the use of alcohol are met as a challenge in a deviation-amplifying process that results in loss of control. Bateson believes that alcohol allows the alcoholic to experience himself as a (complementary) part of the social system, something he cannot do without alcohol. He suggests that AA's philosophy is such that, when perceived in cybernetic terms, it short-circuits the process that pushes the alcoholic to drink and allows him to remain sober, as long as he attends AA. The alcoholic shifts from competitive symmetrical relationships, battling against those who try to get him to stop drinking, to the complementary noncompetitive ones of AA where members define themselves as equally "weak" alcoholics.

Bateson argues that the first step of AA, the recognition of ones' powerlessness over alcohol contradicts the symmetrical pride of the alcoholic without using alcohol. However, the context in which uncontrollable drinking is adaptive looks different if some of the experimental data is examined. This data, and the functioning of the alcoholic in his family of origin suggest an alternative explanation to Bateson's.

Experimental evidence indicates that many alcoholics do not get relief when they drink, even initially, and in fact they feel worse (McGuire et al., 1968; Tamerin et al., 1970). It has been found under experimental conditions that alcoholics, when drinking, become progressively more dysphoric, anxious, agitated and depressed, with the emergence of suicidal agitation (Steinglass, Weiner & Mendelson, 1971), and lower self-esteem (Vanderpool, 1969). Alcoholic "craving," (which as Mello, [1975] states is a tautology), cannot be understood as an attempt to feel better, and can perhaps be perceived as a way to validate bad feelings (Schwartzman, 1985).

A number of experimental studies and detailed clinical descriptions indicate that rather than pride, uncomfortable dependence and/or lack of differentiation appears to be the core problem at least for a number of alcoholics (Blane, 1968; Bowen, 1974). Consequently the functioning and success of AA can be understood, not as a change in epistemology as suggested by Bateson (1971), Kurtz (1982) and others, but in fact as a way of validating their basic premises. The alcoholic's sobriety is maintained by accepting the alcoholics' covert basic premises and altering the definition of the problem to "pride," so that staying the same is the solution, within a context that eliminates alcohol, but allows "slips," and only requires acceptance of the beliefs of AA for membership, making failure impossible.

Schwartzman (1985) has outlined a systemic description of its functioning. The core premise of Alcoholics Anonymous is that group welfare takes precedence over that of the individual, so that personal anonymity is the "spiritual foundation of the fellowship of Alcoholics Anonymous." This is manifest in a number of ways. The officers have ambiguous roles, serve for short periods, and there are no professionals. Members introduce themselves by their first names and describe themselves as alcoholics, validating their equality in their lack of control over alcohol. Much of the content in meetings is the members' self-revelation as alcoholics, discussion of the basic premises of AA and testimony to the solution provided by AA, based on the acceptance of one's alcoholism.

At a more inclusive level, the autonomy of the group is also emphasized. Each group is self-supporting and takes no public positions, except the stated beliefs of Alcoholics Anonymous. The functioning of the group attempts to resolve the problems of dependence and intimacy by the elimination of the self as nearly as possible, defined as "pride." Sobriety and the group are maintained contingent on the loss of individuality, but accompanied by the elimination of conflict and competition.

The famous Twelve Steps — the liturgy of Alcoholics Anonymous — is an isomorph at the level of ideology to that of the "Twelve Traditions" at the level of social structure of the group. The first three steps state that the alcoholic is powerless over alcohol, and should place himself in the power of god, "however conceived," defined so ambiguously as to include almost anything. At a more abstract level, the directive is, "Accept without question that you are acted upon," an analogue to what would be expected as a deutero-learned premise in the alcoholic's family context, and manifest in the alcoholic's behavior and experience as lacking control. This is the opposite message that the alcoholic hears from his significant others, that he should struggle to control his drinking, which generally results in his failing, guilt and humiliation, leading to more drinking, and the amplification of the guilt. Steps Four through Seven suggest a critical self-assessment by which the alcoholic again defines himself as weak, and flawed, rather than fighting this definition. Steps Eight and Nine state that the alcoholic should make amends after an honest personal inventory, so that the alcoholic does not have to respond to his guilt and the amplification of resentments, often used as excuses to continue drinking, leading to more humiliation and alcohol. Instead they suggest a response with appropriate behavior that breaks the pattern. The Twelfth step is to carry the message to other alcoholics as a crucial aspect of one's sobriety, so that the group is self-maintaining.

Davis (1980) notes the similarities between AA and family therapy and suggests how they might be mutually reinforcing. He states that stopping the drinking should always be the first goal in family treatment. In general family therapists agree with this (Bepko, 1985).

TREATMENT OF SUBSTANCE ABUSE

The most successful study of the family therapy of drug abuse remains Stanton et al.'s (1982) study of the structural/strategic brief therapy approach to families with a member addicted to heroin based on the work of Minuchin (1974) and Haley (1980). They assumed the young adult addicts regulated their parents' marriages by their own lack of control, e.g., addiction, and at the same time family constraints short-circuit the addict's developmental process. They together create a self-regulating system in which addiction becomes a means of legitimating lack of change when change is appropriate during the life-cycle. Stanton's group's goal was to put the parents in charge of encouraging the addict's autonomy and recreating the appropriate hierarchy, in terms of expectations and consequences for deviation from appropriate behavior, using basic structural-strategic techniques. This work is one of a very few outcome studies of the efficacy of family therapy for substance abusers using a control group and experimental design. They assessed the families in terms of drug-free days, employment and school attendance and found that paid family therapy was the most effective modality when compared to unpaid family therapy, individual counseling and paid family movies.

Stanton (1979) in a review article, found 68 studies of family treatment of substance abuse with a wide variation, e.g., from multiple outpatient family therapy to inpatient. Of these, only six present outcome of treatment data. Four studies report positive outcomes. There are a number of current studies attempting to measure the efficacy of a similar approach with adolescent drug abusers with less severe drug histories.

One of the problems in the treatment of opiate addiction is that although many treatment facilities overtly accept a systemic family treatment perspective, it is questionable how important this approach is in the actual treatment. There is evidence that those facilities which utilize systemic approaches, often do so only as a peripheral aspect of treatment (Coleman & Stanton, 1978) and/or use therapists minimally trained in family therapy (Coleman & Stanton, 1978).

One of the difficulties in treatment is that substance abuse often becomes part of a more inclusive system that includes treatment facilities, medical personnel, previous therapists, etc. There is evidence that the macrosystems in which many methadone clients interact in the natural history of their treatment are characterized by ambiguous rules and expectations, chronic covert and overt conflict between and within facilities, lack of appropriate transitions, and coalitions between clients and staff. All of these function to create analogues to many of the families of the clients, including chronically addicted members (Schwartzman & Bokos, 1978; Schwartzman, n.d.). In the ongoing study of a methadone clinic, the author found that the lack of clear terminations, unexpressed conflict, and confused hierarchies, created a system analogous to the families of the clients, including their chronicity. In this system, similar processes took place, at a number of levels of organization, in which conflict among those in the system when it reaches a certain level, adds others to the system, and creates another level with the same structure. It seems likely that analogous processes take place in alcohol treatment as they do in the treatment of opiate addicts. Some recent articles have conceptualized more inclusive systems created by all those involved with families with an alcoholic member (Davis, 1980; Schwartzman, 1985; Schwartzman, n.d.; Miller, 1984). Miller has described how those treating alcoholic families are often either incorporated as an impotent ally, or excluded. Consequently, a crucial aspect of theory-building must consider the macrosystemic as a core of treatment (Hunt & Azren, 1973; Ward & Faillace, 1972; Pattison et al., 1975). It must include the family, all those involved in present and past treatment, and awareness of the conflicting beliefs about addiction because these larger systems are always created in treatment, and can create the same pathologies as the families they treat.

At a yet more inclusive level, a number of cultures and subcultures have employed a wide variety of belief systems, rituals, and other institutions to restrict the use of drugs, within tolerable limits, perhaps more successfully than contemporary treatment.

FUTURE RESEARCH, THEORY BUILDING

Pattison and Kaufman (1981) suggest that there are no specific approaches to family treatment of alcoholism, except the necessity of the therapist being active and present-oriented. No study has demonstrated the need for abstinence for effective therapy, although many family therapists state that this is necessary.

Pattison (1977) believes behavioral techniques using "natural stimuli" and cognitive elements of family members offer the most promise for successful treatment. Orford and Edwards (1977) state that natural forces should be utilized in planning therapeutic interventions. Perhaps even more important is the finding by Vaillant (1983), that none of the treatments were more effective than the natural history of alcoholism itself, in which ". . . patients changed life circumstances rather than clinic intervention as most important to their abstinence" (Gerard/Sanger, 1966, in Vaillant, 1983). His own prospective study did not include family therapy. Although a strong advocate, Vaillant admits, ". . . the effectiveness of Alcoholics Anonymous has not been adequately assessed" (Beekland et al., 1975). As he stated: " . . . most of outcome variance in alcohol treatment can be explained by variation in premorbid social stability" (Vaillant 1983, p. 188). In addition, he found that abstaining alcoholics commonly used alternative compulsions, e.g., religious groups, work, other less dangerous drugs, food, cigarettes (Vaillant, 1983, p. 164). At the same time, it has been stated that, ". . . the maintenance of abstinence, the basis for the AA approach, may not represent a reintegration, but rather a condition maintained by continued treatment" (Patteson, 1966, p. 62).

The above discussion suggests that the linearity of the disease model needs to be confronted by the empirical evidence which questions it. A systemic perspective has not been adequately introduced into the field of family treatment of substance abuse, especially treatment of alcoholism. Family therapists have too readily accepted the "conventional wisdom" uncritically in terms of directly confronting denial and insisting on attendance in self-help groups as the primary intervention and abstinence as the only goal. Family interventions in substance abuse are not very imaginative. The direct approach in confronting denial is not necessarily the only or best means to achieve abstinence, since there are few controlled studies or evidence for outstanding therapeutic effectiveness. In addition, since the effectiveness of self-help groups is unclear (Vaillant, 1983), too many family therapists make it the core of their treatment (Bepko, 1985), especially since alcoholics vary in characteristics for which various treatments "fit" (Pattison, 1977), and AA seems to work best for a particular subpopulation (Bean, 1975).

A number of therapists have questioned whether alcoholism is one syndrome, with the same systemic function requiring the same approach. There is evidence that abstinence need not be the only goal of treatment since a number of studies have suggested the possibility of controlled drinking by alcoholics (Davis, 1962). This is the most controversial aspect of alcoholism treatment.

More generally, theories of addiction must ultimately include their cultural and epistemological context. This is not just a question of philosophical inquiry. As stated above, if these levels are not included, the therapeutic systems involved in treatment, self-help groups, and family therapy together, often create a system analogous to that of the families of many of the clients, at a more inclusive level, that seems to maintain the problem. Contradictory goals of treatment create a macrosystem without clear expectations and constraint among those providing treatment, validating lack of control, and reinforcing client's problems.

The maintenance of the pharmacological fallacy by many providing treatment still remains a problem, in that the properties of drugs are described as a given rather than seen in relationship to their context, which is contradicted by experimental, clinical and cultural evidence. This clouds an understanding of larger clinical issues.

REFERENCES

Adler, N. (1972). *The underground stream*. New York: Harper and Row.

Alcohol and Drug Problems Association of North America (1974). National certification of non-professional alcoholism counselors, a report. *ADAP* Washington, DC.

Backeland, F., Lundwall, L. & Kissan, B. (1975). Methods for the treatment of chronic alcoholism: a critical appraisal. In R. J. Gibbons, Y. Isreal, H. Kalant et al. (Eds.), *Research advances in Alcohol and Drug Problems, Vol. 2.* New York, John Wiley & Sons, p. 247-327.

Bales, R.F. (1946). Cultural differences in rates of alcoholism. *Quarterly J Studies on Alcohol, 6*, 482-492.

Bateson, G. (1971). The cybernetics of 'self': A theory of alcoholism. *Psychiatry, 34*, 1-18.

Bateson, G. (1972). *Steps to an ecology of mind*. New York: Ballantine.

Bean, M. (1975). Alcoholics Anonymous. *Psychiatric Annals, 5*, 5-63.

Becker, J.Y. & Miller P.M. (1976). Verbal and nonverbal marital interaction patterns of alcoholics and nonalcoholics. *J Stu Alcohol, 37*, 1616-1624.

Beckman, L.J. (1975). Women alcoholics: A review of the social and psychological studies *J for the Stud on Alcohol, 36*(7), 797-824.

Bennett, L. A., Wolin, S. & McAvity, J. K. (n.d.). Family identity, ritual, and myth: A cultural perspective on life-cycle transitions. In C. Falicov (Ed.), *Family transitions*. Rockville, MD: Aspen Corp.

Bennett, L. A. & Wolin, S. J. (1984). The cross-generational transmission of alcoholism in families: the alcoholism and heritage study. *Anaoli Kinicke bolinice-Dr. M. Stojanovic, 23*, 207-214.

Bepko, C. (1985). *The responsibility trap*. New York: The Free Press.

Bepko, C., (1985). Alcoholism as oppression: The woman in the alcoholic system. In M. Ault-Riche (Ed.), *Women in family therapy*. Rockville, MD: Aspen Corp., p. 64-77.

Blanc, H. (1968). *The personality of the alcoholic*. New York: Harper and Row.

Berenson, D. (1976). Alcohol and the family system. In P. J. Guerin, (Ed.), *Family therapy*. New York: Gardner Press.

Billings, A. G., Kessler, M., Gomberg, C. A. & Weiner, S. (1979). Marital conflict resolution of alcoholic and nonalcoholic couples during drinking and nondrinking sessions. *J Stud Alc, 40*, 183-195.

Bowen, M. (1974). Alcoholism as viewed through family system theory and family psychotherapy. *Annals of the New York Academy of Science, 233*, 115-122.

Calahan, D., Cisin, I. H. & Crossley, H. M. (1969). *American drinking practices: A national study of drinking behavior and attitudes*. New Brunswick: Rutgers Center of Alcoholism Studies.

Calahan, D. & Room, R. (1972). Problem drinking among men age 21-59. *Amer J Public Health, 62*, 1472-1482.

Coleman, S. B. & Stanton, D. M. (1978). Family therapy and drug abuse: A national survey. *Family Process, 17*(1), 21-31.

Coleman, S. B. & Stanton, M. D. (1978). The role of death in the family of the addict. *J Marr Fam, 4*(1), 79-92.

Cork, R. M. (1969). *The forgotten children*. Toronto: Addict. Res. Found.

Cotton, C. S. (1979). The familial incidence of alcoholism. *J Studies on Alcoholism, 40*, 89-116.

Davis, D. I. (1962). Normal drinking recovered alcoholic addicts. *Q J Studies on Alcohol, 23*, 94-104.

Davis, D. I. (1980). Alcoholics anonymous and family therapy. *The J of Marital and Family Therapy, 6*(1), 65-74.

Davis, D. I. & Klagsbrun (1977). Substance abuse and family interaction. *Family Process, 16*(2), 149-178.

Davis, P. I., Berenson, D., Steinglass, P. & Davis, S. (1974). The adaptive consequences of drinking. *Psychiatry, 37*, 209-215.

Diethelm, Y. & Barr, R. M. (1962). Psychotherapeutic interviews and alcoholic intoxication. *Q J Stud Alcohol, 23*, 243-251.

Drewery, J. & Rae, A. B. (1969). A group comparison of alcoholic and nonpsychiatric marriages using the interpersonal perception technique. *Br J of Psychiatry, 115*, 287-300.

Edwards, H., Harvey, C. & Whithead, P. C. (1973). Wives of alcoholics: A critical review and analysis. *Q J Stu Alcohol, 34*, 112-132.

El-Guebly, N. & Offord, D. R. (1977). The offspring of alcoholics: A critical review. *Amer J of Psy, 134*, 357-365.

Edwards, P., Harvey, C. & Whitehead, P. C. (1973). Wives of alcoholics: A critical view and analysis. *Q J Stud Alcohol, 34*, 112-132.

Ewing, J. A. & Fox, R. I. (1968). Family therapy and alcoholism. In J. Masserman (Ed.), *Current Psychiatric therapies, Vol. 8*, New York: Grune and Stratton.

Foy, D., Miller, P. & Eisler, R. (1979). *The effects of alcohol consumption on the marital interactions of chronic alcoholics*. San Francisco: Assoc. Adv. Behavior Therapy.

Fox, R. (1962). Children in the alcoholic family. In W. C. Bier (Ed.), *Problems in addiction: Alcohol and drug addiction*. New York: Fordham University Press.

Ganger, R. & Schugart, G. (1966). The heroin addict's pseudoassertive behavior and family dynamics. *Soc Casework, 47*, 643-649.

Gerard, G. L. & Saenger, G. (1966). Outpatient treatment of alcoholism: A study of outcome and its determinants. Toronto, *Brookside Monograph #4*.

Gerard, D. L., Saegner, G. & Wile, R. (1962). The abstinent alcoholic. *Arch Gen Psy, 6*, 83-95.

Gillis, L. S. & Keet, M. (1969). Prognostic factors and treatment results in hospitalized alcoholics. *Q J Studies in alcohol, 30*, 426-437.

Gomberg, E. S. (1981). Women, sex roles and alcohol problems. *Professional Psychology, 12*, 146-155.

Goodwin, D. W. (1985). Alcoholism and genetics. *Arch Gen Psych, 42*, 171-174.

Gorad, S. L. (1971). Communicational styles and interaction of alcoholics and their wives. *Family Process, 10*, 475-589.

Haley, J. (1980). *Leaving home*. New York: McGraw-Hill.

Hoffman, H. & Noem, A. A. (1975). Alcoholism among patients of male and female alcoholics. *Psycho Reports, 36*, 332-348.

Hunt, G. M. & Azrin, N. H. (1973). A community-reinforcement approach to alcoholism. *Beh Res and Therapy, 11*, 91-111.

Hyman (1976). Alcoholics 15 years later. *Annals of the New York Academy of Science, 273*, 613-623.

Jackson (1956). The adjustment of the family to alcoholism. *Marr Family, 18*, 361-369.

Jacob, T., Favorini, A., Meisel, S. S. & Anderson, C. M. (1978). The alcoholic's spouse, children and family interaction: Substantive findings and methodological issues. *J Stud Alcoh, 39*, 1231-1251.

Jaffe, J. (1972). Cited in R. Glasscote, J. Sussex, J. Ball, & L. Brill. *The treatment of drug abuse*. Washington, DC: American Psychiatric Association.

Jellinck (1960). *The disease concept of alcoholism*. New Haven: Hillhouse Press.

Jones, M. C. (1968). Personality correlates and antecedents of drinking patterns of behavior in adult males. *J Consult Clin Psy, 32*, 2-12.

Jones, M. C. (1971). Personality antecedents and correlates of drinking patterns in women. *J Consult Clin Psychol, 35*, 61-69.

Kandel, D. B., Kessler, R. C. & Margulies, R. S. (1978). Antecedents of adolescents, initiation into stages of drug use: A developmental analysis. *J of Youth & Adolescence, 7*(1), 13-14.

Kaufman, E. (1985). Commentary on Steinglass et al., *Family Process, 24*, 377-379.

Kaufman, E. (1985). *The power to change*. New York: Gardner Press.

Kaufman, E. & Kaufmann, P. (1978). *The family therapy of drug and alcohol abusers*. New York: Gardner Press.

Kaufman, E. & Pattison, M. (1981). Differential methods of family therapy in the treatment of alcoholism. *J Stud Alco, 40*, 1-29.

Kuhn, T. (1962). *The theory of scientific revolution*. Chicago: University of Chicago Press.

Kurtines, W. M., Ball, L. R. & G. H. Wood (1978). Personality characteristics of long-time recovered alcoholics: A comparative analysis. *J Consulting and Clinical Psychology, 46*, 971-977.

Kurtz, E. (1979). *Not-God: A history of alcoholics anonymous*. Center City, MN: Hazelden.

Kurtz, E. (1982). Why AA works: The intellectual significance of alcoholics anonymous. *J Stud Alcohol, 43*, 38-80.

Liebson, I. A., Bigelow, G. & Flamer, R. (1973). Alcoholism among methadone patients: A specific treatment method. *Amer J Psy, 130*, 483-485.

Ludwig, A. M. (1972). On and off the wagon: Reasons for drinking and abstaining by alcoholics. *Q J Stu Alc, 33*, 91-96.

MacAndrew, C. & Edgerton, R. (1969). *Drunken deportment: A social explanation*. Chicago: Aldine.

McClelland, D. C., Davis, W. N. & R. Kahn (1972). *The drinking man*. New York: The Free Press.

Mcguire, M. T., Mendelson, J. H. & Stein, S. (1966). Comparative psychosocial studies of alcoholic and nonalcoholic subjects undergoing experimentally-induced ethanol intoxication. *Psychosomat Med, 28*, 13-26.

McNamee, H. B., Mello, N. K. & Mendelson, J. T. (1968). Experimental analysis of drinking patterns of alcoholics: Concurrent psychological observations. *Am J Psychiatry, 124*, 1063-1068.

Mardones, J. (1963). The alcohols. In W. S. Root & F. G. Hoffman (Eds.), *Physiological pharmacology*. New York: Academic Press, pp. 89-103.

Marshall, M. (1979). *Beliefs, behaviors, and alcoholic beverages*. Ann Arbor: University of Michigan Press.

Meeks, D. & Kelley, C. (1970). Family therapy with the families of recovering alcoholics. *Q J Stud Alc, 31*(2A), 399-413.

Mello, N. (1975). A semantic aspect of alcoholism. In A. D. Chappel & A. E. LeBlan (Eds.), *Biological and behavioral approaches to drug dependence*. Toronto: Alcoholism and Drug Research Foundation, pp.73-87.

Merry, J. (1966). 'The loss of control' myth. *Lancet, 1*, pp. 1257-1258.

Miller, D. (1983). Outlaws and invaders: The adaptive function of alcohol abuse in the helper-supra system. *J of Strategic and Systemic Therapies, 2*(3), 15-27.

Minuchin, S. (1974). *Families and family therapy*. Cambridge, MA: Harvard University Press.

Nathan, P. E., Goldman, M. S., Lisman, S. A. & Taylor, H. A. (1972). Alcohol and alcoholics: A behavioral approach. *Transactions New York Academy of Sciences, 34*, 602-627.

Olsen, D. & Killerin, N. E. (1984). Chaotic flippers in treatment. In E. Kaufman (Ed.), *Power to change*. New York: Gardner Press.

Orford, J. (1975). Alcoholism and marriage: The argument against specialism. *J Stud Alc*, 1537-1563.

Orford, J. & Edwards, G. (1977). *Alcoholism*. New York: Oxford University Press.

Paredes, A., Hood, W. R., Seymour, H. & Gollum, M. (1973). Loss of control in alcoholism: An investigation of the hypothesis with experimental findings. *Q J of Studies on Alcohol, 34*, 1146-1161.

Pattison, E. M.'(1965). Treatment of alcoholic families with nurse home visits. *Family Process, 4*, 74-94.

Pattison, E. M. (1966). A critique of alcoholism treatment concepts, with special reference to abstinence. *Q J Stud Alcohol, 27*, 49-71.

Pattison, E. M. (1977). Ten years of change in alcoholism treatment and delivery systems. *Amer J of Psy, 134*(3), 261-266.

Pattison, E. M., DeFrancisco, D., Frazier, H. et al., (1975). A psychosocial kinship model for family therapy. *Amer J Psych, 132*(12), 1251-1257.

Pattison, E. M. & Kaufman, E. (1981). Family therapy and the treatment of alcoholism. In M. R. Lansky (Ed.), *Family therapy and major psychopathology*. New York: Grune and Stratton.

Paulino, R. & McCready, B. (1977). *The alcoholic marriage: Alternative perspectives*. New York: Grune and Stratton.

Pettinati, H. M. (1981). Carrier foundation: Following alcoholics for four years. *Carrier Foundation Letter, 70*, 1-4.

Poole, S. (1985). The cultural context of psychological approaches to alcoholism. *American Psychologist, 39*(12), 1337-1351.

Rimmer, J. & Winokur, G. (1972). The spouses of alcoholics: An example of assortive mating. *Dis Nerv System, 33*, 509-511.

Room, R. (1977). Measurement and distribution of drinking patterns and problems in general populations. In G. Edwards et al. (Eds), *Alcohol Related Disabilities*. WHO Offset Publication No. 32. Geneva: World Health Organization.

Schuckit, M. A., Pitts, F. N., Reich, T., King L. J. & Winokur, G. (1969). Two types of alcoholism in women. *Arch Gen Psy, 20*, 321-326.

Schwartzman, J. (1975). The addict, abstinence and the family. *Amer J Psy, 132*(2), 154-157.

Schwartzman, J. (1983). Ritual, change, and psychotherapy. *Australian J of Psychotherapy, 4*(3), 159-163.

Schwartzman, J. (1985). Alcoholics anonymous and the family: A systemic perspective. *Amer J Drug Alcohol Abuse, 11*(1&2), 69-89.

Schwartzman, J. (n.d.) The natural history of a drug treatment system.

Schwartzman, J. & Kroll, L. (1977). Addict abstinence and methadone maintenance. *International J of the Addictions, 12*(4), 497-507.

Schwartzman, J. & Bokos, P. (1979). Methadone maintenance: The addict's family recreated. *International J of Family Therapy*, 338-355.

Scott, E. M. (1970). *Struggles in an alcoholic family*. Springfield: Charles C. Thomas & Sons.

Stanton, M. D. (1977). The addict as savior: Heroin, death and the family. *Family Process, 16*, 191-197.

Stanton, M. D. (1979). Family treatment approaches to drug abuse problems: A review. *Family Process, 18*(3), 251-280.

Stanton, M. D. & Todd, T. (1982). *The family therapy of drug abuse and addiction*. New York: Guilford Press.

Steinglass, P. (1976). Experimenting with family treatment approaches to alcoholism 1950-1975: A review. *Family Process, 24*(4), 97-123.

Steinglass, P. (1980). A life history model of the alcoholic family. *Family Process, 19*(3), 211-226.

Steinglass (1985). Rejoinder: The clinician verses the statistician. *Family Process, 24*(3), 380-383.

Steinglass, P., Weiner, S. & Mendelsion, J. H. (1971). International issues as determinants of alcoholism. *Am J Psychiatry, 128*, 275-280.

Steinglass, P. & Tislenko, Reiss, D. (1985). Stability/instability in the alcoholic marriage. *Family Process, 34*(30), 365-376.

Syme, L. (1957). Personal characteristics and the alcoholic: A critique of current studies. *Q J Stud Alcohol, 18*, 288-302.

Tamerin, J. S., Weiner, S. & Mendlson, J. H. (1970). Alcoholic's expectancies, and recall of experiences during intoxication. *Am J Psychiatry, 126*, 1696-1704.

Tarter, R. E. (1976). Personality of wives of alcoholics. *J Clin. Psych, 32*(30), 741-743.

Trice, H. M. (1958). Alcoholics anonymous. *Ann Amer Acad Pol Soc Sci, 315*, 108-116.

Trice, H. M. & Roman, P. M. (1970). Sociopsychological predicators of affiliation with alcoholics anonymous: A longitudinal study of treatment success. *Social Psychiatry, 5*, 51-59.

Vaillant, G. (1966). A 12-year follow-up of New York addicts, IV: Some characteristics and determinants of abstinence. *Amer J Psych, 123*, 573-584.

Vaillant, G. (1983). *The natural history of alcoholism*. Cambridge: Harvard University Press.

Vanderpool, J. A. (1969). Alcoholism and the self concept. *Q J Stu Alcohol, 30*, 59-77.

Walsh, F. (1978). Concurrent grandparent death and birth of schizophrenic offspring an intriguing finding. *Family Process*, *17*, 457-473.

Ward, R. F. & Faillace, L. A. (1970). The alcoholic and his helpers: A systems view. *Q J Stud of Alco*, *31*, 684-691.

Wolin, S. J., Bennett, L. & Noonan, D. L. (1979). Family rituals and the occurrence of alcoholism over the generations. *Am J Psy*, *136*, 589-593.

Wolin, S. J., Bennett, L. A., Noonan, D. L. & Teitelbaum, M. A. (1980). Disrupted family rituals: A factor in the intergenerational transmission of alcoholism. *J of the Studies on Alcohol*, *41*, 199-241.

Ziegler-Driscoll, G. (1979). The similarities in families of drug dependents and alcoholics. In E. Kaufman & P. Kaufmann (Eds.), *Family therapy of drug and alcohol abuse*. New York: Gardner Press.

Families and Chronic Medical Illness

Peter Steinglass
Mary Elizabeth Horan

In 1962, Meyer and Haggerty published a paper reporting findings from a study examining the relationship between family stress and susceptibility to streptococcal infection. One hundred (100) individuals from a total of 16 lower-middle class families were followed for a 12-month period during which time throat cultures were taken every three weeks, and whenever an acute infection occurred. Their rather provocative findings indicated that the incidence of clinical streptococcal infections in members of the families studied could not be predicted simply by knowing whether or not the throat culture results were positive. In fact, in over 50% of the cases where beta-hemolytic streptococci were isolated on throat culture, no concurrent clinical infection was present. Further, there was no significant association of streptococcal illness with such host-related variables as sex, family history of repeated infections, strong personal allergic history, the presence or absence of tonsils, or even family size. That is, none of these factors seemed to account for the differential outcome regarding clinical infection in instances when throat cultures were positive.

Instead, the incidence of clinical infections was most strongly associated with a very different type of "challenge" — an episode of acute family stress, as measured by interview and diary data about the occurrence of life events that had disrupted family life. If one compared the time period two weeks before and two weeks after the onset of a streptococcal infection, an acute family crisis was *four times* more likely to have occurred during the pre-illness time period than the two weeks post-illness. Further, fully one-quarter of all clinical infections

The authors are affiliated with Center for Family Research, George Washington University School of Medicine, Washington, DC 20037.

The preparation of this paper was supported by Rehabilitation Research and Training Center Grant G008300123 from the National Institute for Handicapped Research (David Reiss, MD, Principal Investigator).

127

were found to have followed such an episode of family stress. Meyer and Haggerty concluded,

> Not only are higher acquisition and illness rates associated with acute and chronic stress situations, but also the proportion of persons in whom there is a significant rise of anti-streptolysin 0 (the antibody level) following the acquisition of streptococci increases with increasing stress. (p. 547)

The Meyer-Haggerty study dealt with a seemingly straightforward medical condition, an infectious disease. The classical biomedical explanation for the "cause" of such a disease points to two factors as primary — an infectious agent and the adequacy of host defense mechanisms. This study suggested a somewhat different conclusion, however. The individual's ability to resist clinical infections seemed to be tied not only to the adequacy of biological defenses (immunological responses) but also to the status of the person's primary social environment (the family).

The Meyer-Haggerty study is merely one of a growing number of studies that could be cited as evidence of the importance of family factors in the onset and course of medical illness. In this paper we want to explore these interrelationships; *first*, by discussing some of the evolving clinical and research perspectives which attempt to establish a place for the family in the understanding of chronic illness, and providing some examples of the types of studies and findings being generated by each of these perspectives, and *second*, by discussing some of the unique challenges faced by family researchers and clinicians working in this area.

FAMILY PERSPECTIVES ON MEDICAL ILLNESS

An overview of the literature on family factors in chronic medical illness indicates that four different perspectives have been represented which we will call, respectively: the "resource" perspective; the "deficit" perspective; the "course" perspective; and the "impact" perspective.

The Family as Resource

This *first* perspective focuses on the family as a resource for the individual in coping with illness. The basic argument here is that the family, as the primary source of social support for its members, both serves a protective or prophylactic role in strengthening individual resistance to illness (a preventive function), and is a major determinant of successful compliance with treatment regimens once medical illness has been diagnosed. Strong support for this position comes from a series of studies indicating that such family qualities such as empathy, and the family's own coping resources have been associated with improvements in medical condition and patient compliance with medical treatment (Litman, 1966; Litman, 1974; Oakes, Ward, Gray, Klauber & Moody, 1970; Patterson & McCubbin, 1983; Robertson & Suinn, 1968). Further, the compelling evidence that social supports are critical in coping successfully with medical illness (Anderson & Auslander, 1980; Anderson, Auslander, Achtenberg & Miller, 1981; Anderson, Miller, Auslander & Santiago, 1983; Greenberg, Weltz, Spitz & Bizzozero, 1975; Pentecost, Zwerenz & Manuel, 1976; Sherwood, 1983; Steidl, Finkelsein, Wexler, Feigenbaum, Kitsen, Kliger & Quinlan, 1980) also establishes the importance of the family (as the primary social support resource for the individual) in this formula.

An example of a study guided by this first perspective is the investigation of diabetic adolescents and their families carried out by Anderson et al. (1981), in which an attempt was made to contrast the family environments of 53 diabetic adolescents in good, fair and poor control. The central finding of this study — that families with diabetic children in good metabolic control, compared to those in poor control, reported less conflict, greater cohesion, more encouragement of self-sufficiency and independence, and greater parental involvement and sharing in the responsibility for diabetes care — is then interpreted as evidence that such a family environment, when available, is a major resource accounting for the positive adjustment of some of these adolescent diabetics. Another way of phrasing such a conclusion is that the availability of a supportive, high-functioning family has a positive effect on clinical outcome. Thus in this formulation the emphasis is clearly on the protective capabilities of the family vis-à-vis the impact of the illness on the patient.

As another example, Steidl and his colleagues (1980), focusing on family factors which might be associated with increased adherence to medical treatment in patients receiving hemodialysis, coded family interaction patterns using a modification of the Beavers-Timberlawn scales applied to videotaped family interaction sessions. They found that patients who complied with the prescribed treatment regimen tended to come from families whose members: (1) negotiate and solve problems efficiently; (2) adhere to the generational boundaries between children and parents; (3) are responsive to one another; and (4) acknowledge their own responsibility for their past and present actions rather than blaming others. Here again, the emphasis is on the ability of the well-functioning family to support its member in efforts to successfully cope with chronic medical illness.

The Psychosomatic Family: A Deficit Model

This second perspective sees the family not as a potential resource, but rather as a potential active contributor to the development of illness. Here the main influence of the family is not so much in protecting its members from illness, but rather in increasing the incidence of illness by debilitating its members secondary to the consequences of a dysfunctional, rigid and stressful family environment. This second perspective has often been called the "deficit" model of family factors in illness.

Although at first glance this second perspective would appear to be merely the flip side of the first, it in fact has generated studies of very different character. Here the family is seen as a negative influence; in the first perspective the family is conceptualized as a buffering agent.

This perspective is perhaps most clearly represented by the pioneering research into the "psychosomatic family" carried out by Salvador Minuchin and his colleagues (Minuchin, Rosman & Baker, 1978; Minuchin, Baker, Rosman, Liebman, Milman & Todd, 1975), but has subsequently been espoused by numerous other investigators and clinicians as well (Bloch, 1984; Grolnick, 1983; Jaffe, 1978; Kogg, Vandereycken & Vertommen, 1985; Malow & Olson, 1984; Penn, 1983; Stierlin, 1983; Zager & Marquette, 1981). The basic conceptual approach in all of these investigations is the same — because families in which there is a chronically ill member seem to share certain structural properties and characteristic response styles, it is hypothesized that these factors are critical in rendering an individual family member susceptible to disease.

As characterized by Minuchin and his colleagues in the classical formulation of the "psychosomatic family," four family characteristics are crucial: (1) enmeshment and overinvolvement of family members as seen in poorly differentiated subsystem boundaries; (2) overprotection of each family member which interferes with the unfolding of the separation individuation process; (3) rigid transactional patterns aimed at maintaining the status quo at all costs; and (4) a lack of conflict resolution in which conflicts are either denied or avoided. Such a family, according to Minuchin et al., presents itself to the outside world as a conflict-free unit whose only concern is the presence of a chronic illness in one of its family members.

Although a number of other investigators have offered important suggestions regarding possible modifications of the Minuchin model—e.g., Stierlin (1983) has proposed that in addition to bound and enmeshed family systems, split and disintegrating family relational patterns similarly impact on the development and maintenance of chronic illness—these modifications can be looked upon as attempts to fine-tune the model; not as fundamental disagreements with the "deficit" perspective toward family factors and chronic medical illness.

Studies adopting this "psychosomatic family" perspective look not only to family characteristics that predispose its members to medical illness but also imply that the family is therefore an *etiologic* agent in the onset of disease. In particular, these studies attempt to identify specific family factors that not only are associated with increased incidence of medical illness, but are also temporally related to the clinical exacerbations of chronic episodic medical conditions like labile diabetes (Crain, Sussman & Weil, 1966; McCord, McCord & Verdon 1960: Minuchin et al., 1978; Pond, 1979), auto-immune diseases (Cobb, Schull & Harburg, 1969; Medsger & Robinson, 1972), chronic pain (psychogenic pain disorder) (Liebman, Honig & Berger, 1976; Malow & Olson, 1984; Mohmed, Weisz & Waring, 1978; Roy, 1982) and classical psychosomatic illness (Block, 1969; Boyce, Jensen, Cassel, Collier, Smith & Ramey, 1977; Engel, 1955: Jackson & Yalom, 1966).

However, the "psychosomatic family" construct remains a controversial one. Some investigators have found it a powerful model for interpreting their research findings; other investigators have critiqued the model as lacking in clear operational definitions of its core dimensions. As an example of a study that has embraced the Minuchin et al., model, Mallow and Olson (1984), using the Family Concept Inventory to compare families of myofascial pain dysfunction (MPD) syndrome patients with non-patient families, found that MPD syndrome patients perceive their families as significantly more involved in each others lives, more ambitious and more concerned with success, prestige, and accomplishments. Mallow and Olson imply that these impressions resemble those qualities of enmeshment, over-protectiveness, rigidity, and lack of conflict resolution which Liebman, Minuchin and Baker (1970) have identified as characterizing families who are faced with other psychophysiologic illnesses.

On the other hand, we have the critique of the Minuchin et al., model offered by Kog and her colleagues (1985). Pointing to the considerable conceptual confusion associated with the four central concepts of the "psychosomatic family" model, Kog et al., contend that existing definitions of these dimensions preclude their operationalization and valid measurement in research designs. For example, they contend that many researchers have confused the Minuchin et al., construct of enmeshment-disengagement with rigidity of family interaction patterns or with a dichotomy in emotional quality of family relationships. When the enmeshment-disengagement dimension is operationalized in such a fashion, it becomes indistinguishable from at least two other dimensions within the model – rigidity and overprotectiveness of the ill family member (when a child).

Kog et al., suggest that the above difficulties might be obviated by redefining the core dimensions of the model. Instead of the four dimensions suggested by Minuchin, they proposed three fundamental interactional dimensions that they label: the intensity of intrafamilial boundaries; the degree of the family's adaptability; and the family's way of handling conflicts. It is their contention that each of these dimensions is ordinally scaled and hence can be effectively operationalized and measured using family interaction or questionnaire methods.

But they would also caution that until such a revision in the Minuchin et al., model is widely adopted, the underlying validity of the model remains largely untested. Thus the substantial body of studies cited above that purport to demonstrate a etiological role for family environmental factors in the development or perpetuation of chronic medical illness must, according to this argument, be viewed with considerable caution because the models the studies use for interpretation of data are conceptually flawed.

Family Influences on the Course of Chronic Illness

The third perspective reflected in the literature on the family and chronic medical illness focuses primarily on the *course* of chronic medical illness. Whereas the first two perspectives dealt with family factors that decrease or increase likelihood of the development of illness (onset) or exacerbation of episodic conditions, this perspective looks at how the family influences the differential course of chronic illness (Bray, 1977; Christopherson, 1962). These studies, as a group, contend that because different illness characteristics and phases place different demands on the family (Rolland, 1984; Stein, 1982), the manner in which the family responds to these challenges may therefore have a profound impact on the individual's adjustment to the illness.

Often operating within a systems perspective, these studies look at the interface between family behavior and illness characteristics and ask questions about how family and illness variables mutually reinforce one another as the illness moves into its chronic phase. Often the question being asked is what aspects of family behavior serve to *maintain* the chronicity of medical illnesses, and vice versa. The systemic implications of such family factors as "exclusionary coalitions" between patient and select family members (Penn, 1983; Sheinberg, 1983) stability of the marital dyad (Kaplan De-Nour & Czaczkes, 1974; Malmquist, 1973; Streltzer, Finkelstein & Feigenbaum, 1976), family communication patterns (Pentecost, Zwerenz & Manuel, 1976), and quality of family daily routines (Boyce et al., 1977; Steinglass, 1981) have all emphasized that specific family patterns seem to be associated with increased chronicity of medical illness.

Impact of Illness on the Family

The fourth and final perspective we want to mention focuses not so much on the way family factors influence the onset or course of chronic medical conditions, but rather on the impact of the illness on the family. Surely chronic medical conditions take their toll on families, draining valuable family emotional, practical and financial resources (Fife, 1980; Maurin & Schenkel, 1976; Patterson & McCubbin, 1983; Satterwhite, 1978; Tarnow & Tomlinson, 1978). Looked at from this perspective, it is the potential impact of the medical illness on the family's overall psychosocial and vocational functioning that should command our attention.

For example, Maurin and Schenkel (1976) interviewed families in which one member with end stage renal failure was being maintained on hemodialysis. Overinvolvement in family (if not patient) life replaced a broader social life. Additionally, while the patient's needs were met, other family members' needs were not attended to. The investigators suggest that the level of over-involvement may lead to serious psychological implications such as unexpressed anger, frustration, and guilt—in other words, powerful documentation and reminders of the profound implications of chronic illness for family life.

Studies within this perspective have also included an interest in illness-related factors that correlate with differential family impacts. An example: Based on parental interviews, school reports and psychological testing of 404 chronically ill children and their families in five separate studies, Satterwhite (1978) found that the impact of an illness on psychosocial aspects of family functioning depended in part on the perceived severity of the illness. Parents identified general worry, finances, fatigue of parent, decreased social life, and change in sleeping arrangements and furnishings as areas of particular concern.

Originally, studies of the impact of chronic illness on the family took a categorical approach to defining the stresses associated with medical illness. That is, studies looked at family impact disease by disease, and potential family stressors were thought to be properties of the specific disease itself. For example, diabetic patients share a common set of characteristics which impact on the families of diabetics. Families of cardiac patients, on the other hand, are faced with a different set of challenges which stem from the cardiac condition itself. Thus we see review articles that focus on a specific disease (e.g., Anderson & Auslander, 1980; Kaplan De-Nour, 1980) rather than on particular types of stresses or impacts.

Underlying this perspective is the assumption that the family is a passive recipient of demands and stresses associated with a particular illness. As an extension of this perspective, a prevailing idea amongst medical social service providers is that only families struggling with the same illness "can understand what we are going through." Consequently, psychosocial services provided by medical treatment facilities are characteristically organized around specific illnesses. Thus the same medical center might have separate family programs for diabetes, cancer, cardiac rehabilitation, etc.

More recently, it has been suggested that a preferable approach is to develop typologies of medical illnesses based on the types of psychosocial challenges presented to all families with chronically ill members (Rolland, 1984; Stein & Jessop, 1982). Here the differential impact on the family would presumably be tied to the qualitative differences between illnesses along each of these generic chronic illness dimensions.

For example, in the Rolland model chronic illnesses are grouped according to commonly shared biological characteristics that dictate significantly different psychosocial challenges for the patient and for the family. Illnesses vary in their onset (acute or gradual), course (progressive, constant or episodic) and degree of incapacitation. Thus, an incapacitating illness characterized by a gradual onset and a progressive course (such as late onset multiple sclerosis. Huntington's chorea or scleroderma) presents considerably different types of stressors to a family than does an acute onset illness (like epilepsy or asthma) which follows a relapsing but non-incapacitating course.

The time phase of an illness (crisis, chronic, or terminal) would be another characteristic that might differentially challenge the family, requiring different strengths, attitudes and changes from the family

(Carter, 1984; Steinglass, Temple, Lisman & Reiss, 1982). The total amount of readjustment of family structure, roles, problem-solving and affective coping might be the same for both types of illness but the manner in which the adjustments occur is qualitatively different.

Thus although struggling with diverse medical conditions, families share common life experiences as a result of the illness. The degree of success with which the family negotiates these challenges and integrates the illness into family life in turn strengthens or weakens the impact of the psychosocial stressors on the family and on the individual's adjustment to the illness.

RESEARCH AND TREATMENT CHALLENGES

Although the clinical literature on families and chronic medical illness is by now quite substantial, it is also the case that most reviewers of this literature have urged caution regarding the conclusions one can draw from existing data. The most frequently mentioned concern is the quality of the research methodology typically encountered in this body of literature.

The vast bulk of investigations concerning family factors and chronic illness employs either case study or correlational designs. Neither of these approaches allows for causal interpretations about the interactive effects between illness and family factors. Thus whether the "resource," "deficit," "course," or "impact" perspectives makes the most sense in approaching this subject remains largely unresolved. Further, sample sizes tend to be small, are usually convenience rather than representative samples, and are rarely evaluated from the perspective of possible cultural or social class biases. There is also the problem of the use of self-report measures (most of the instruments currently in use to assess adjustment to illness and family impact use a self-report format). Self-report measures have long been considered somewhat suspect as accurate reflections of specific illness-related behaviors such as compliance with medical regimen or incidence of physical symptoms.

However, many of the above concerns are not specific to family-chronic illness studies, but rather are generic to the study of the family, and hence are raised whenever family studies are being reviewed. But there are also a number of issues that are unique to the area of family factors and chronic medical illness. We see three such challenges as of particular relevance to the family-oriented clinician and hence will discuss them further at this point.

"Normal" vs. "Pathological" Responses to Chronic Medical Illness

A working assumption in much of the research done to date is that traditional measures of psychopathology and psychosocial distress are appropriate and valid indices of maladaptation to medical illness. Yet a number of investigators have contended that such symptoms as depression and anxiety are ubiquitous in chronic illness patients, especially those dealing with debilitating diseases. Further, the growing evidence that denial is not only one of the most commonly used defense mechanisms for coping with illness, but may also in certain instances be a highly adaptive defense, means that any attempt to draw conclusions about adequacy of adaptation by interviewing patients alone may be fraught with danger.

Suppose, for example, a study seems to demonstrate that psychiatric symptom levels in chronic dialysis patients, determined via use of a traditional symptom checklist like the SCL-90, are very low. Should we conclude from such a study that dialysis has an insignificant impact on people's psyches? Or should we instead see in these data evidence of widespread denial of symptoms amongst such patients? Or might we even conclude that the challenges of dialysis bring out the best in people and such a population is therefore composed of super-copers?

One attempt to remedy this dilemma has been the development of a new generation of research measures designed specifically for use with medical illness populations. An example is the Psychological Adjustment to Illness Scale (PAIS) (Morrow, Chiarello & Derogatis, 1978). This scale asks respondents to report on adequacy of adjustment in seven areas of functioning thought to be particularly relevant measures of level of coping with chronic medical illness — health care orientation, vocational environment, domestic environment, sexual relationships, extended family relationships, social environment, and psychological distress. Such instruments offer considerable promise, but are still in limited use. Hence norms have not yet been firmly established, and it is still unclear whether separate norms will have to be developed for different types of illnesses (using either a categorical or Rolland-type model for identifying illness categories).

Biology vs. Psychology

Many chronic medical illnesses have direct effects on the central nervous system, often producing profound cognitive and emotional disturbances. Such disturbances occur not only when the disease is one that directly affects the CNS (e.g., brain tumors, CVAs, multiple sclerosis), but also when the condition produces metabolic imbalances that impede brain functioning (e.g., diabetes, renal failure, cirrhosis). In such instances it is often extremely difficult, if not impossible, to determine whether evidence of psychosocial distress is functional in origin, or a side effect of organic disturbances created by the disease process itself. Errors can occur in both directions, with organicity misinterpreted as evidence of functional psychosis/character pathology, or psychological distress (especially depression) falsely attributed to a metabolic imbalance. In such situations, therefore, it is critical that studies include careful measures of both psychological and medical status. Hence research teams must have both types of expertise represented.

Yet another factor is extremely important in this regard. It is also the case that modern, high technology medical treatments are themselves associated with profound psychological challenges. For example, specific psychiatric syndromes have been associated with CCU and ICU treatments (Hackett, Cassem & Wishnie, 1968; McKegney, 1966), and many of the pharmacological protocols currently in use for treating chronic medical conditions (e.g., chemotherapy) have numerous CNS side effects. In such instances it is critical that psychological response patterns be seen as iatrogenic in origin, and not be interpreted as evidence of the fragility of coping mechanisms. Hence in such a situation the normative response pattern may be to develop anxiety, depression, disorientation, and perhaps even psychotic symptoms. How to define a "pathological" response pattern in such a situation then becomes highly problematic, further complicating the selection of adequate criteria of "healthy" adjustment.

Patient Health vs. Family Health

Another major challenge, and one with profound implications for treatment, is that it is not always clear that what is best for the patient is also best for the family. That is, it is entirely possible that a treatment plan thought to be ideal for successful management of a particular chronic medical condition might itself be a source of stress for the family. For example, home hemodialysis might substantially improve the patient's sense of psychological independence and work productivity, but at the same time place vastly greater demands on other family members regarding dialysis responsibilities. In this sense the patient's increased mobility is achieved at the expense of the family's overall mobility.

As another example, home care for a seriously disabled post-CVA patient may be associated with significantly less depression and increased motivation for rehabilitation, but might also mean increased financial drain for the family, the need to redesign living space within the home, disruption of family routines, and alteration of family priorities (Steinglass, Temple, Lisman & Reiss, 1982). In such an instance, stabilization of the patient's medical and psychological status may be accompanied by the emergence of significant distress and psychopathology in another family member, a member who was previously symptom-free. In the Steinglass, Temple, Lisman and Reiss (1982) paper, a case example is described in which a family had devoted itself to the home care of a spinal cord injured patient and had been so "successful" at it that they were often cited by the medical team as an example of how families can best cope with spinal cord injury. However, a careful family history revealed that two of the three children in the family were experiencing significant developmental difficulties, marked deterioration in school performance and evidence of significant depression. Further, the family had had no vacations since the traumatic injury to the husband/father, and when they finally attempted to arrange a vacation that didn't include the patient, he experienced a dramatic deterioration in functioning, became psychotically depressed, and within two months of the vacation had died.

A similar picture emerges in the data recently reported by Reiss and his colleagues (Reiss, Gonzalez & Kramer 1986) from a study of family factors associated with differential course of end stage renal disease (ESRD) patients on chronic hemodialysis. In this study of 23 families, each with an ESRD patient, meticulous assessments were carried out of three family attributes thought to be potential resources for positive coping with chronic illness — family problem-solving strategies as assessed via performance on a standardized laboratory family problem-solving task; family intelligence and overall level of accomplishment assessed via traditional questionnaire measures; and family intactness indicated by measures of duration of the marriage and presence of living grandparents. These measures were then compared with two measures of "successful coping" with the illness — degree of compliance with the medical regimen; and whether the patients were alive or dead at two-year follow-up.

The most dramatic and surprising finding was that those families who were judged to be better problem-solvers (higher scores on variables previously ascertained as associated with positive functional indices), had higher mean IQ and family accomplishment scores, and greater level of intactness were also families in which the index patient had died by the time of follow-up assessment. This association was so strong that a discriminant function analysis, using the family variables to predict whether the index patient was alive or dead at follow-up, correctly classified all 23 cases.

A second major finding, which was equally unanticipated, was that *noncompliance* with the medical regimen (measured via weight fluctuation between dialysis sessions, serum phosphorus levels, and nurse ratings) was highly correlated with *survival*, not death of the index patients. Further, noncompliance seemed to be a major "mediating" variable between the family factors and survival (as indicated via partial-order correlational analyses).

Presented with a clinical situation such as the spinal cord injury family described above, it often appears that the clinician is faced with the choice of whether to place the health needs of the patient center stage, or to design a program intended to maximize family psychological health. The dramatic findings reported by Reiss and his colleagues can only heighten this clinical dilemma.

A CONCLUDING STATEMENT: IMPLICATIONS FOR FAMILY THERAPY

Although a perspective that sees the family as a resource for the medically ill individual would appear to suggest that patient health and family health are synonymous, the unique demands associated with the illness and its ideal medical treatment often conflict with critical family functions. As was documented in our review of the literature, chronic medical illness often becomes an organizing principle for family life, with concomitant distortions in family development and alterations in family regulatory processes. In such cases, the family's attempts to cooperate with the medical team and follow instructions regarding the treatment plan inadvertently undermines family health.

Thus chronic medical conditions also present unique challenges to the family therapist in the design of interventions that respect not only the psychological health of the family, but also ensure that the patient's medical treatment is being adequately supported. Our own efforts to meet this challenge (Steinglass, Gonzalez, Dosovitz & Reiss, 1982; Gonzalez, Steinglass & Reiss, 1986) have centered around the design and implementation of a short-term multiple-family discussion group (MFDG) approach that borrows heavily from principles utilized in psychoeducational programs for chronic psychiatric disorders (e.g., see Anderson, Reiss & Hogarty, 1986). An eight-session treatment in which four to six families with a chronically ill member (heterogeneous regarding medical condition) meet weekly to discuss issues of shared relevance, this particular MFDG uses as its central metaphor the need to "find a place for the illness within the family, while at the same time ensuring that the illness is kept in its place." Three major components — an educational, family issues (problem-solving), and feelings (affects) component — are addressed by the families in an effort to define those aspects of family life that seem *generic* to the chronic illness issue and those coping styles that families find most helpful in dealing with the stresses associated with the illness.

Clearly, family therapy approaches to chronic medical illness are still in their infancy. However, it is already apparent that success in this area will not come from a simple extension of traditional methods to the problems associated with medical conditions, but instead will demand new approaches that build carefully on the growing body of findings from family research, findings that underscore how unique and often counterintuitive are the conclusions to be drawn in this area.

REFERENCES

Anderson, B. J. & Auslander, W. F. Research on diabetes management and the family: A critique. *Diabetes Care*, 1980, *3*(6), 696-702.

Anderson, C.M., Reiss, D.J. & Hogarty, G. E. *Schizophrenia and the family.* 1986, New York: Guilford Press.

Anderson, B. J., Auslander, W. F., Achtenberg, J. & Miller, J. P. Impact of age and parent-child and spouse responsibility sharing in diabetes management on metabolic control. *Diabetes*, 1983, *32*, 17A.

Anderson, B. J., Miller, J. P., Auslander, W. F. & Santiago, J. V. Family characteristics of diabetic adolescents: Relationship to metabolic control. *Diabetes Care*, 1984, *4*, 586-594.

Bloch, D. A. The family as a psychosocial system. *Family Systems Medicine*, 1984, *2*(4), 387-396.

Block, J. Parents of schizophrenic, neurotic, asthmatic and congenitally ill children. *Archives of General Psychiatry*, 1969, *20*, 659-674.

Boyce, W. T., Jensen, E. W., Cassel, J. C., Collier, A. M., Smith, A. H. & Ramey, C. T. Influence of life events and family routines on childhood respiratory tract illness. *Pediatrics*, 1977, *60*(4), 609-615.

Bray, G. Reactive patterns in families of the severely disabled. *Rehabilitation Counseling Bulletin*, 1977, March, 236-239.

Carter, R. E. Family reactions and reorganization patterns in myocardial infarction. *Family Systems Medicine*, 1984, *2*(1), 55-65.

Christopherson, V. The patient and the family. *Rehabilitation Literature*, 1962, February, 34-41.

Cobb, S., Schull, W. J., Harburg, E. & Kasl, S. V. The intrafamilial transmission of rheumatoid arthritis: An unusual study. *Journal of Chronic Diseases*, 1969, *22*, 193-194.

Crain, A. J., Sussman, M. B. & Weil, W. B. Effects of a diabetic child on marital integration and related measures of family functioning. *Journal of Health and Human Behavior*, 1966, *7*, 122-127.

Engel, G. L. Studies of ulcerative colitis. *American Journal of Medicine*, 1955, *19*, 232-256.

Falloon, I.R.H., Boyd, J.L. & McGill, C.W. *Family Care of Schizophrenia.* 1984, New York: Guilford Press.

Fife, B. L. Childhood cancer is a family crisis: A review. *Journal of Psychiatric Nursing*, 1980, *18*(10), 29-39.

Gonzalez, S., Steinglass, P. & Reiss, D. *Family-centered interventions for the chronically disabled: The eight-session multiple-family discussion group program. Treatment manual.* 1986, Washington, DC: George Washington University Rehabilitation Research and Training Center.

Greenberg, I. M., Weltz, S., Spitz. C. & Bizzozero, J. Factors of adjustment in chronic hemodialysis patients. *Psychosomatics*, 1975, *16*(4), 178-184.

Grolnick, L. Ibsen's truth, family secrets, and family therapy. *Family Process*, 1983, *22*(3), 797-797.

Hackett, T.P., Cassem, N.H. & Wishnie, H.A. The coronary care unit: Appraisal of its psychological hazards. *New England Journal of Medicine*, 1968, *279*, 1365-1370.

Jackson, D. D. & Yalom, I. Family research in the problem of ulcerative colitis. *Archives of General Psychiatry*, 1966, *15*, 410-418.

Jaffe, D. T. The role of family therapy in treating physical illness. *Hospital and Community Psychiatry*, 1978, *29*, No. 3, 169-174.

Kaplan De-Nour, A. Dialysis within the context of the family. *International Journal of Family Psychiatry*, 1980, *1*, 61-75.

Kaplan De-Nour, A., & Czaczkes, J.W. Team-patient interaction in chronic hemodialysis units. *Psychotherapy and Psychosomatics*, 1974, *24*, 132-136.

Kliger, A. S. & Quinlan, D. M. Medical condition, adherence to treatment regimens, and family functioning. *Archives of General Psychiatry*, 1980, *37*, 1025-1027.

Kog, E., Vandereycken, W. & Vertommen, H. The psychosomatic family model. A critical analysis of family interaction concepts. *Journal of Family Therapy*, 1985, *7*, 31-44.

Liebman, R., Minuchin, S. & Baker, I. The use of structural family therapy in the treatment of intractable asthma. *American Journal of Psychiatry*, 1970, *131*, 535-540.

Liebman, R., Honig, P. & Berger, H. An integrated treatment program for psychogenic pain. *Family Process*, 1976, *15*, 397-405.

Litman, T. J. The family and physical rehabilitation. *Journal of Chronic Diseases*, 1966, *19*, 211-217.

Litman, T. J. The family as a basic unit in health and medical care: A social-behavioral overview. *Social Science and Medicine*, 1974, *8*(9-10), 495-519.

Mallow, R. M. & Olson, R. E. Family characteristics of myofascial pain dysfunction. *Family Systems Medicine*, 1984, *2*(4), 428-431.

Malmquist, A. A prospective study of patients in chronic hemodialysis – I. Method and characteristics of the patient group. *Journal of Psychosomatic Research*, 1973, *17*, 333-337.

Maurin, J. & Schenkel, J. A study of the family unit's response to hemodialysis. *Journal of Psychosomatic Research*, 1976, *20*(3), 163-168.

McCord, W., McCord, J. & Verdon, P. Familial correlates of psychosomatic symptoms in male children. *Journal of Health and Human Behavior*, 1960, *1*, 192-199.

McKegney, F. P. Intensive care syndrome: Definition, treatment and prevention of a new "disease of medical progress." *Connecticut Medicine*, 1966, *30*, 633-636.

Medsger, A. & Robinson, H. A comparative study of divorce in rheumatoid arthritis and other rheumatoid diseases. *Journal of Chronic Diseases*, 1972, *25*, 269-275.

Meyer, R. J. & Haggerty, R. J. Streptococcal infections in families. Factors altering individual susceptibility. *Pediatrics*, 1962, *29*, 539-549.

Minuchin, S., Baker, L., Rosman, B. L., Liebman, R. Milman, L., & Todd, T.C. A conceptual model of psychosomatic illness in children. *Archives of General Psychiatry*, 1975, *32*, 1031-1038.

Minuchin, S., Rosman, B.L. & Baker, L. *Psychosomatic Families*. 1978. Cambridge, MA: Harvard University Press.

Mohamed, S. J., Weisz, G. M. & Waring, E. M. The relationship of chronic pain to depression, marital adjustment and family dynamics. *Pain*, 1978, *5*, 285-292.

Morrow, G.R., Chiarello, R.J. & Derogatis, L.R. A new scale for assessing patients' psychosocial adjustment to medical illness. *Psychological Medicine*, 1978, *8*, 605-610.

Oakes, T. W., Ward, J. R., Gray, R. M., Klauber, M. R. & Moody, P. M. Family expectations and arthritis patient compliance to a hand-resting splint regimen. *Journal of Chronic Diseases*, 1970, *22*, 757-764.

Patterson, J. M. & McCubbin, H. I. Chronic illness: Family stress and coping. In C. F. Figley & H. I. McCubbin (Eds.), *Stress and the Family. Volume II: Coping with Catastrophe*. New York: Brunner/Mazel, 1983.

Penn, P. Coalitions and binding interactions in families with chronic illness. *Family Systems Medicine*, 1983, *1*(2), 16-25.

Pentecost, R. L., Zwerenz, B. & Manuel, J. W. Intrafamily identity and home dialysis success. *Nephron*, 1976, *17*, 88-103.

Pond, H. Parental attitudes toward children with a chronic medical disorder: Special reference to diabetes mellitus. *Diabetes Care*, 1979, *2*(5), 425-31.

Reiss, D., Gonzalez, S. & Kramer, N. Family process, chronic illness and death. *Archives of General Psychiatry*, 1986, *43*(8), 795-807.

Robertson, E. K. & Suinn, R. M. The determination of rate of progress of stroke patients through sympathy measures of patient and family. *Journal of Psychosomatic Research*, 1968, *12*, 189-191.

Rolland, J. S. Toward a psychosocial typology of chronic and life-threatening illness. *Family Systems Medicine*, 1984, *2*(3), 245-262.

Roy, R. Marital and family issues in patients with chronic pain. *Psychotherapy and Psychosomatics*, 1982, *37*, 1-12.

Satterwhite, B. B. Impact of chronic illness on child and family: An overview based on five surveys with implications for management. *International Journal of Rehabilitation Research*, 1978, *1*, 7-17.

Sheinberg, M. The family and chronic illness: A treatment diary. *Family Systems Medicine*, 1983, *1*, 26-36.

Sherwood, R. J. Compliance behavior of hemodialysis patients and the role of the family. *Family Systems Medicine*, 1983, *1*(2), 60-72.

Steidl, J. H., Finkelstein, F. O., Wexler, J. P., Feigenbaum, H., Kitsen, J., Kliger, A. S. & Quinlan, D. M. Medical condition, adherence to treatment regimens, and family functioning. *Archives of General Psychiatry*, 1980, *37*, 1027-27.

Stein, R. E. & Jessop, D. J. A noncategorical approach to chronic childhood illness. *Public Health Report*, 1982, *97*(4), 354-362.

Steinglass, P. The alcoholic family at home. *Archives of General Psychiatry*, 1981, *38*, 578-584.

Steinglass, P., Gonzalez, S., Dosovitz, I. & Reiss, D. Discussion groups for chronic hemodialysis patients and their families. *General Hospital Psychiatry*, 1982, *4*, 7-14.

Steinglass, P., Temple, S., Lisman, S. A. & Reiss, D. Coping with spinal cord injury: The family perspective. *General Hospital Psychiatry*, 1982, *4*, 259-264.

Steirlin, H. Family therapy—A science or an art? *Family Process*, 1983, *22*(4), 413-23.

Streltzer, J., Finkelstein, F. & Feigenbaum, H. The spouse's role in home dialysis. *Archives of General Psychiatry*, 1976, *33*(1), 55-58.

Tarnow, J. D. & Tomlinson, N. Juvenile diabetes: Impact of the child and family. *Psychosomatics*, 1978, *19*(80), 487-491.

Zager, R. P. & Marquette, C. H. Developmental considerations in children and early adolescents with spinal cord injury. *Archives of Physical Medical Rehabilitation*, 1981, *62*, 427-431.

Family Systems and Chronic Illness: A Typological Model

John S. Rolland

INTRODUCTION

This paper will offer a conceptual base for theory building, clinical practice, and research investigation in the area of chronic and life-threatening illness. This model should furnish a central reference point from which clinicians and researchers of different persuasions may forge their own trails.

For clinicians and researchers alike, the heart of all systems-oriented biopsychosocial inquiry is the focus on *interaction*. In the arena of physical illness, particularly chronic disease, one's focus of concern is the system created by the interaction of a disease with an individual, family or other biopsychosocial system (Engel, 1977, 1980). From the family point of view, family systems theory must include the illness system in its thinking. A graphic representation of the family/illness system created by the interface of a family facing chronic disease might look like that depicted in Figure 1.

There are critical missing links in this preliminary description of the dynamic interaction between these two systems. First, there is a need for a schema that recasts the myriad of biological diseases into psychosocial terms. Second, refinement and expansion of a general family systems model is needed to allow a more appropriate and comprehensive description of the interactive system created when chronic illness occurs in the family. This paper will address the first issue. A psychosocial typology of illness and time phase model will be described so that a more fluid dialogue can occur between the illness aspect and family aspect of the illness/family system.

John S. Rolland, MD, is Medical Director, Center for Illness in Families, New Haven, CT, and Assistant Clinical Professor, Department of Psychiatry, Yale University School of Medicine.

This paper is a revised and expanded version of one that originally appeared in *Family Systems Medicine* (Rolland, 1984).

INTERFACE OF CHRONIC ILLNESS AND THE FAMILY

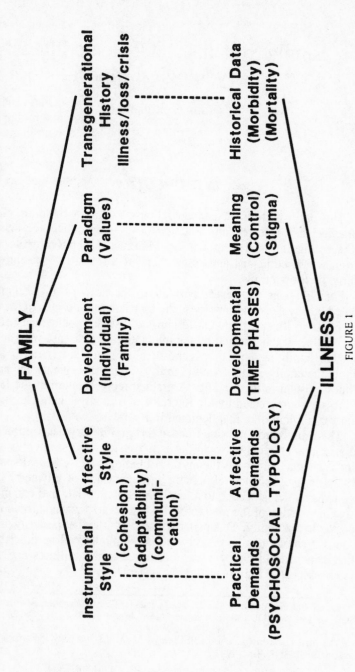

FIGURE 1

In order to think in an interactive or systemic manner about the interface of the illness and the individual or the illness and the family, one needs a way of characterizing the illness itself. A schema to conceptualize chronic diseases is required that remains relevant to the interactions of the psychosocial and biological worlds and provides a common meta-language that transforms or reclassifies the usual biological language. Such a schema will facilitate coherent thinking about the system created at the interface of chronic illness with many other systems. However, there are two major impediments to progress in this area. First, insufficient attention has been given to the areas of diversity and commonality inherent in different chronic illnesses. Second, there has been a glossing over of the qualitative and quantitative differences in how various diseases manifest themselves over the time course of the illness. Chronic illnesses need to be conceptualized in a manner that organizes these similarities and differences over the disease course so that the type and degree of demands relevant to psychosocial research and clinical practice are highlighted in a more useful way.

Before proposing a solution, let us examine the origins of the problem more closely. The great variability of chronic illnesses and their changing nature over time have presented a vexing problem to psychosocial investigators who have attempted to identify the most salient psychosocial variables relevant to disease course or treatment compliance. Recent reviews of the psychosocial modifiers of stress emphasize a variety of methodological and conceptual weaknesses (Elliot & Eisdorfer, 1982; Kasl, 1982; Weiss et al., 1981). The difficulty originates when social scientists or psychotherapists accept a disease classification that is based on purely biological criteria that are clustered in ways to meet the needs of medicine. This nosology fits the world of anatomy, physiology, biochemistry, microbiology, physical diagnosis, pharmacology, surgery, etc. From a traditional medical point of view, the diagnosis of a specific illness is of primary concern because it dictates subsequent treatment planning. One can argue that the problem of psychosocial research in physical illness suffers as much from a blind acceptance of this unshakable model of medicine as from its own shortcomings. We hinder progress in clarifying the relationship of psychosocial factors to disease course if we limit ourselves to a biological framework that categorizes information to diagnose and treat illness from a biological perspective.

Historically, this specific illness orientation has guided research and clinical investigations of the relationship between psychosocial factors and physical illness toward opposite ends of a continuum. Truths are sought either in each specific illness or in "illness" as a general, sometimes metaphorical, concept. This can lead to two types of problems. Findings with one disease are then generalized to cover all illnesses indiscriminately. Or, findings are held to be not generalizable and researchers study each illness in a narrow-focused way. Both of these extremes hamper the clinician. Because of a lack of guidelines to balance unifying principles and useful distinctions, clinicians can become bewildered by the wide variety of chronic illnesses. They may apply a monolithic treatment approach to all chronic illnesses. They may inappropriately transpose aspects of their clinical experience with psychiatric disorders. Extensive experience with a single kind of illness that requires intensive focus on issues of separation and loss, like terminal cancer, may get transferred to a chronic illness, like stroke, where other issues such as role reallocation predominate.

The psychosocial importance of different time phases of an illness is another dimension that is not well understood. A major reason for this in research has been the relative predominance of cross-sectional, in contrast to longitudinal, studies. Often, studies include cases that vary widely in terms of the amount of time families have lived with a chronic illness (Atcherberg et al., 1977; Blumberg et al., 1954; Turk, 1964). Often, separate investigations of the same disease produce conflicting results. Debates ensue without either side taking into account the factor of time phase as a plausible explanation for the different results. Likewise, clinicians often become involved in the care of an individual or family coping with a chronic illness at different points in the "illness life cycle." Clinicians rarely follow the interaction of a family-illness through the complete life history of a disease.

A few studies have explored short-range psychosocial effects on disease course. One study noted a synchronicity of emotional and behavioral factors with joint tenderness ratings in individuals with rheumatoid arthritis (Modolfsky & Chester 1970). Others have studied diabetic and asthmatic exacerbations (Minuchin et al., 1975; Baker et al., 1975; Bradley, 1979; Hamburg et al., 1980; Matus & Bush, 1979). Minuchin, in his classic study with children with brittle diabetes, used the accepted medical correlation between a rise in blood serum free fatty-acid levels and the development of diabetic ketoacidosis. He demonstrated a sustained rise of serum levels when the children were introduced into an interview where the parents were discussing a conflictual issue. Although these studies are important, their contributions concern microfluctuations rather than broad scale phases of an illness (crisis, chronic, end stage or terminal).

The importance of broad time phases of illness has surfaced periodi-

cally in the chronic illness literature. One example is the role of denial
at different points of the disease course. For parents of a child with
leukemia, denial may enable them adaptively to perform necessary
duties during earlier phases of the illness, but might lead to devastating consequences for the family if maintained during the terminal
phase (Chodoff et al., 1964; Wolff et al., 1964). Likewise, denial may
be functional for recovery on a coronary care unit after a myocardial
infarction, but harmful if this translates into ignoring medical advice
vis-à-vis diet, exercise and work stress over the long term (Croog et
al., 1971; Hackett et al., 1968). Again, these studies highlight the
importance of a longitudinal perspective (in this instance in relation to
a particular defense mechanism—denial), but an overarching framework is not articulated.

There is an obvious need for a conceptual model that will provide a
guide useful to both clinical practice and research, one that allows a
dynamic open communication between these disciplines. The first section of this paper proposes a typology of chronic or life-threatening
illness. The problems of illness variability and time phases are addressed on two separate dimensions: (1) chronic illnesses are grouped
according to key biological similarities and differences that dictate
significantly distinct psychosocial demands for the ill individual and
his/her family; (2) the prime developmental time phases in the natural
evolution of chronic disease are identified. In the second part of the
paper, I will discuss some of the clinical, research, and health services
delivery implications of this schema.

PSYCHOSOCIAL TYPOLOGY OF ILLNESS

Any typology of illness is by nature arbitrary. The goal of this typology is to facilitate the creation of categories for a wide array of
chronic illnesses. This typology is designed not for traditional medical
treatment or prognostic purposes, but to examine the relationship between family or individual dynamics and chronic disease.

This typology conceptualizes broad distinctions of (1) onset, (2)
course, (3) outcome, and (4) degree of incapacitation of illness. These
categories are hypothesized to be the most significant at the interface
of the illness and the individual or family for a broad range of diseases. Also, there is a correspondence between each of the categories:
onset, course and outcome, and a particular temporal phase of chronic
disease. While each variable is in actuality a continuum, it will be
described here in a categorical manner by the selection of key anchor
points along the continuum.

Onset

Illnesses can be divided into those which have either an acute or gradual onset. This division is not meant to differentiate types of biological development, but to distinguish the kinds of symptomatic presentation that can be noted by the patient subjectively or other individuals objectively. Strokes and myocardial infarction are examples of illnesses with sudden clinical presentation, but arguably long periods of biological change that led to a marker event. Examples of gradual onset illnesses include arthritis, emphysema and Parkinson's disease. For an illness with gradual onset, like rheumatoid arthritis, the diagnosis serves as a somewhat arbitrary confirmation point after clinical symptoms have started.

A gradual crisis presents a different form of stressor to an individual or family than a sudden crisis. The total amount of readjustment of family structure, roles, problem solving and affective coping might be the same for both types of illness. However, for acute onset illnesses, like stroke, these affective and instrumental changes are compressed into a short time. This will require of the family more rapid mobilization of crisis management skills. Some families are better equipped to cope with rapid change. Families able to tolerate highly charged affective states, exchange clearly defined roles flexibly, problem solve efficiently and utilize outside resources will have an advantage managing acute onset illnesses.

The rate of family change required to cope with gradual onset diseases, like rheumatoid arthritis or Parkinson's disease, allows for a more protracted period of adjustment while perhaps generating more anxiety before a diagnosis is made. For acute onset diseases, there is relatively greater strain on the family to juggle their energy between protecting against further disintegration, damage or loss through death, and progressive efforts that maximize mastery through restructuring or novel problem solving (Adams & Lindemann, 1974).

Course

The course of chronic diseases can take essentially three general forms: progressive, constant, or relapsing/episodic. A *progressive* disease (e.g., cancers, Alzheimer's disease, juvenile onset diabetes, rheumatoid arthritis and emphysema) by this definition is one that is continually or generally symptomatic and progresses in severity. The individual and family are faced with the effects of a perpetually symptomatic family member, where disability increases in a stepwise or progressive fashion. Periods of relief from the demands of the illness tend to be minimal. Continual adaptation and role change is implicit. Increasing strain on family caretakers is caused by both the risks of exhaustion and the continual addition of new caretaking tasks over time. Family flexibility both in terms of internal role reorganization and their willingness to use outside resources are at a premium.

It is profitable to distinguish further between illnesses that progress rapidly or slowly. The demands on the family coping with a rapidly progressive illness such as nonresponsive lung cancer or acute leukemia are different than the demands of slowly progressive illnesses like rheumatoid arthritis, chronic obstructive pulmonary disease (e.g., emphysema, chronic bronchitis), or adult onset diabetes. The pace of adaptation required to cope with the continual changes and ever new demands of a rapidly progressive disease mounts as the time course shortens. A slowly progressive illness may place a higher premium on stamina rather than continual adaptation.

A *constant* course illness is one where typically an initial event occurs after which the biological course stabilizes. Examples include: stroke, single-episode myocardial infarction, trauma with resulting amputation or spinal cord injury with paralysis. Typically, after an initial period of recovery, the chronic phase is characterized by some clearcut deficit such as paraplegia, amputation, speech loss or a cognitive impairment. Or, there may be a residual functional limitation like a diminished physical stress tolerance or a restriction of previous activities. Recurrences can occur, but the individual or family is faced with a semipermanent change that is stable and predictable over a considerable time span. The potential for family exhaustion exists without the strain of new role demands over time.

The third kind of course is characterized as *relapsing* or *episodic*. Illnesses like ulcerative colitis, asthma, peptic ulcer, migraine headaches and multiple sclerosis are typical. Forms of cancer in remission, such as resectable and chemotherapy responsive kinds, might be included in this category. The distinguishing feature of this kind of disease course is the alternation of stable periods of varying length, characterized by a low level or absence of symptoms, with periods of flare-up or exacerbation. Often the family can carry on a "normal" routine. However, the specter of a recurrence hangs over their heads.

Relapsing illnesses demand a somewhat different sort of family adaptability. Relative to progressive or constant course illnesses, they may require the least ongoing caretaking or role reallocation. But, the episodic nature of an illness may require a flexibility that permits movement back and forth between two forms of family organization. In a sense, the family is on-call to enact a crisis structure to handle exacerbations of the illness. Strain on the family system is caused by both the frequency of transitions between crisis and noncrisis, and the ongoing uncertainty of *when* a crisis will next occur. Also, the wide psychological discrepancy between periods of normalcy versus illness is a particularly taxing feature unique to relapsing chronic diseases.

Outcome

The extent to which a chronic illness is a likely cause of death and the degree to which it can shorten one's life span is a critical distinguishing feature with profound psychosocial impact. The most crucial factor is the *initial expectation* of whether a disease is a likely cause of death. On one end of the continuum are illnesses that do not typically affect the life span such as, lumbosacral disc disease, blindness, arthritis, spinal cord injury or seizure disorders. At the other extreme are illnesses that are clearly progressive and usually fatal such as metastatic cancer, A.I.D.S., and Huntington's chorea. There is an intermediate more unpredictable category. This includes both illnesses which shorten the life span such as cystic fibrosis, juvenile onset diabetes and cardiovascular disease, and those with the possibility of sudden death such as hemophilia, or recurrences of myocardial infarction or stroke.

All chronic illnesses potentially involve the loss of bodily control, one's identity, and intimate relationships (Sourkes, 1982). For a life-threatening illness the loss of control entails greater consequences — death and the permanent loss of relationships. The ill member fears life ending before living out his/her "life plan" and of being alone in death. The family fears becoming survivors alone in the future. For both there exists an undercurrent of anticipatory grief and separation that permeates all phases of adaptation. Families are often caught between a desire for intimacy and a pull to "let go" emotionally of the ill member. The future expectation of loss can make it extremely difficult for a family to maintain a balanced perspective. A literal torrent of affect could potentially distract a family from the myriad of practical tasks and problem solving that maintain family integrity (Weiss, 1983). Also, the tendency to see the ill family member as practically "in the coffin" can set in motion maladaptive responses that divests the ill member of important responsibilities. The end result can be the structural and emotional isolation of the ill person from family life. This kind of psychological alienation has been associated with poor medical outcome in life-threatening illness (Davies et al., 1973; Derogatis et al., 1979; Schmale & Iker, 1971; Simonton et al., 1980).

For illnesses that may shorten life or cause sudden death, loss is less imminent or certain an outcome than for clearly fatal and nonfatal illnesses. Because of this, issues of mortality predominate day-to-day life less. It is for this reason that this type of illness provides such a fertile ground for idiosyncratic family interpretations. The "it could happen" nature of these illnesses creates a nidus for both over-protection by the family and powerful secondary gains for the ill member. This is particularly relevant to childhood illnesses such as hemophilia, juvenile onset diabetes and asthma (Minuchin et al., 1975, 1978).

Incapacitation

Incapacitation can result from impairment of cognition (e.g., Alzheimer's disease), sensation (e.g., blindness), movement (e.g. stroke with paralysis, multiple sclerosis), energy production and disfigurement or other medical causes of social stigma. Illnesses such as cardiovascular and pulmonary diseases impair the body's ability to produce raw energy. This can lower peak performance or the ability to sustain motor, sensory or cognitive efforts. Illnesses such as leprosy, neurofibromatosis or severe burns are cosmetically disabling to the extent that sufficient social stigma impairs one's ability for normal social interaction.

The different kinds of incapacitation imply sharp differences in the specific adjustments required of a family. For instance, the combined cognitive and motor deficits of a person with a stroke necessitate greater family role reallocation than a spinal cord injured person who retains his/her cognitive faculties. Some chronic diseases like hypertension, peptic ulcer, many endocrine disorders, or migraine headache cause either none, mild or only intermittent incapacitation. This is a highly significant factor moderating the degree of stress facing a family. For some illnesses, like stroke or spinal cord injury, incapacitation is often worst at the time of onset and would exert its greatest influence at that time. Incapacitation at the beginning of an illness magnifies family coping issues related to onset, expected course, and outcome. For progressive diseases, like multiple sclerosis, rheumatoid arthritis or dementia, disability looms as an increasing problem in later phases of the illness. This allows a family more time to prepare for anticipated changes. In particular, it provides an opportunity for the ill member to participate in disease-related family planning.

As a caveat, several studies cite the importance of the family's expectations of a disabled member. An expectation that the ill member could continue to have responsible roles and autonomy was associated with both a better rehabilitation response and successful long-term integration into the family (Bishop & Epstein, 1980; Cleveland, 1980; Hyman, 1975; Litman, 1974; Slater et al., 1970, Sussman & Slater, 1971; Swanson & Maruta, 1980). Bishop and Epstein (1980) envisioned that the family would have the greatest difficulty in deciding realistic role expectations with both mildly disabling illnesses, which were most ambiguous in their demands, and the most severely incapacitating ones because of the sheer amount of role change required.

In sum, the net effect of incapacitation on a particular individual or family depends on the interaction of the type of incapacitation with the pre-illness role demands of the ill member and the family's structure and flexibility. However, it may be the presence or absence of *any* significant incapacitation that constitutes the principal dividing line relevant to a first attempt to construct a psychosocial typology of illness (Viney & Westbrook, 1981).

By combining the kinds of onset (acute versus gradual), course (progressive versus constant versus relapsing/episodic), outcome (fatal versus shortened life span versus non-fatal) and incapacitation (present versus absent) into a grid format we generate a typology with 32 potential psychosocial types of illness. It is clear that certain types of disease (i.e., constant course fatal illnesses) are so rare or non existent that for practical purposes they can be eliminated. This grid is shown in Figure 2. The number of potential types can be reduced further by combining or eliminating particular factors. This would depend on the relative need for specificity in a particular situation.

The extent to which illnesses are predictable has not been formulated as a separate category in the typology. Rather, predictability should be seen as a kind of metacharacteristic that overlays and colors the other attributes: onset, course, outcome and incapacitation.

There are two distinct facets to the predictability of a chronic illness. Diseases can be more or less uncertain as to the *actual* nature of the onset, course, outcome, or presence of incapacitation. And, they can vary as to the *rate* at which changes will occur. Some diseases like spinal cord injury can be accurately typed at the point of diagnosis and have a highly predictable course. Other illnesses such as stroke, myocardial infarction, hypertension or lung cancer are rather unpredictable as to course and outcome. With these kinds of diseases the initial prediction of type may change. For instance, if a second episode occurs, a stroke or myocardial infarction can be considered relapsing or progressive. Lung cancer can become incapacitating if brain metastases occur. Some cases of lung cancer progress rapidly. Others advance slowly with a long remission, or not at all ("spontaneous cure"). Some illnesses like rheumatoid arthritis or migraine headaches

		INCAPACITATING ACUTE	INCAPACITATING GRADUAL	NONINCAPACITATING ACUTE	NONINCAPACITATING GRADUAL
PROGRESSIVE	F A T A L		Lung cancer with CNS metastases A.I.D.S. Bone marrow failure Amyotrophic lateral sclerosis	Acute leukemia Pancreatic cancer Metastatic breast cancer Malignant melanoma Lung cancer Liver cancer, etc.	Cystic fibrosis *
RELAPSING				Cancers in remission	
PROGRESSIVE	P O S S I B L Y F A T A L / S H O R T E N E D L I F E S P A N		Emphysema Alzheimer's disease Multi-infarct dementia Multiple sclerosis (late) Chronic alcoholism Huntington's chorea Scleroderma		Juvenile diabetes * Malignant hypertension Insulin dependent adult onset diabetes
RELAPSING		Angina	Early multiple sclerosis Episodic alcoholism	Sickle cell disease * Hemophelia *	Systemic lupus erythematosis *
CONSTANT		Stroke Mod/severe myocardial infarction	P.K.U. and other inborn errors of metabolism	Mild myocardial infarction Cardiac Arrhythmia	Hemodialysis treated renal failure Hodgkins disease
PROGRESSIVE	N O N F A T A L		Parkinson's disease Rheumatoid arthritis Osteo-arthritis		Non-insulin dependent adult onset diabetes
RELAPSING		Lumbosacral disc disease		Kidney stones Gout Migraine Seasonal allergy Asthma Epilepsy	Peptic ulcer Ulcerative colitis Chronic bronchitis Other inflam. bowel diseases Psoriasis
CONSTANT		Congenital malformations Spinal cord injury Acute blindness Acute deafness Survived severe trauma & burns Post-hypoxic syndrome	Non-progressive mental retardation Cerebral palsy	Benign Arrhythmia Congenital heart disease	Malabsorption syndromes Hyper/Hypothroidism Pernicious anemia Controlled hypertension Controlled glaucoma

* early

FIGURE 2. Categorization of Chronic Illnesses by Psychosocial Type. Reprinted by permission from *Family Systems Medicine*, 2:3, pp. 245-262.

tend to have predictable long-range courses, but can be highly variable day to day. This kind of uncertainty can interfere more with daily rather than long-term planning. The typology of illness cannot predict these changes. In a particular case, if important changes occur during the course of the disease, an individual can switch from one illness type to another.

Several other important attributes that differentiate illnesses were excluded from this typology because they seemed of lesser importance or were relevant to only a subgroup of disorders. When appropriate they should be considered in a thorough systemically-oriented evaluation. The complexity, frequency and efficacy of a treatment regimen, the amount of home versus hospital based care required by the disease, and the frequency and intensity of symptoms vary widely across illnesses and have important implications for individual and family adaptation. Finally, the age of illness onset in relation to child, adult and family stages of development is a critical factor beyond the scope of this paper (Rolland, 1987).

TIME PHASES

To complete a matrix, the time phases of an illness need to be considered as a second dimension. Often one hears about "coping with cancer," "managing disability," or "dealing with life-threatening illness." These cliches can create a kind of tunnel vision, that precludes sufficient attention to the phases of an illness. Each phase has its own psychosocial tasks which require significantly different strengths, attitudes, or changes from a family. To capture the core psychosocial themes in the natural history of chronic disease, three major phases can be described: (1) crisis, (2) chronic, and (3) terminal. The relationship between a more detailed chronic disease time line and one grouped into broad time phases can be diagrammed as depicted in Figure 3.

The *crisis* phase includes any symptomatic period before actual diagnosis when the individual or family has a sense something is wrong, but the exact nature and scope of the problem is not clear. It includes the initial period of readjustment and coping after the problem has been clarified through a diagnosis and initial treatment plan.

During this period, there are a number of key tasks for the ill member and his/her family. Moos (1984) describes certain universal practical illness related tasks. These include: (1) learning to deal with pain, incapacitation or other illness-related symptoms; (2) learning to deal with the hospital environment and any disease-related treatment procedures and; (3) establishing and maintaining workable relationships with the health care team. In addition there are critical tasks of a more general, sometimes existential nature. The family needs to: (1) create a meaning for the illness event that maximizes a preservation of a sense of mastery and competency; (2) grieve for the loss of the pre-

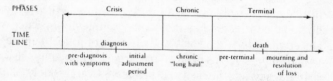

FIGURE 3. Time Line and Phases of Illness. Reprinted by permission from *Family Systems Medicine*, 2:3, pp. 245-262.

illness family identity; (3) move toward a position of acceptance of permanent change while maintaining a sense of continuity between their past and future; (4) pull together to undergo short-term crisis reorganization and; (5) in the face of uncertainty develop a special system flexibility toward future goals.

The *chronic* phase can be long or short, but essentially it is the time span between the initial diagnosis and readjustment period and the third phase when issues of death and terminal illness predominate. It is an era that can be marked by constancy, progression or episodic change. In this sense, its meaningfulness cannot be grasped by simply knowing the biological behavior of an illness. Rather it is more a psychosocial construct, that has been referred to as "the long haul," or "day-to-day living with chronic illness" phase. Often the individual and family has come to grips psychologically and/or organizationally with the permanent changes presented by a chronic illness and has devised an ongoing modus operandi. At one extreme, the chronic phase can last for decades as a stable, nonfatal chronic illness. On the other hand, it may be nonexistent in an acute onset, rapidly progressive fatal disorder where the crisis phase is contiguous with the terminal phase. The ability of the family to maintain the semblance of a normal life under the "abnormal" presence of a chronic illness and heightened uncertainty is a key task of this period. For a fatal illness, it is a time of "living in limbo." For certain highly debilitating not clearly fatal illnesses, such as a massive stroke or dementia, the family can become saddled with an exhausting problem "without end." Paradoxically, some families' hope to resume a "normal" life cycle might only come through the death of their ill member. This highlights another crucial task of this phase: the maintenance of maximal autonomy for *all* family members in the face of a pull toward mutual dependency and caretaking.

The last phase is the *terminal* period. It includes the preterminal stage of an illness where the inevitability of death becomes apparent and predominates family life. It encompasses the periods of mourning and resolution of loss. It is the predominance of issues surrounding separation, death, grief, resolution of mourning, and resumption of "normal" family life beyond the loss that distinguishes this phase.

Beyond their own significance, the three phases illuminate critical transition points linking each period. Apt descriptions in the adult development and family life cycle literature have clarified the importance of transition periods (Levinson, 1978; Carter & McGoldrick, 1980). It is the same for the transitions between developmental phases in the course of disease. This is a time of reevaluation of the appropriateness of the previous family life structure in the face of new illness-related developmental demands. Unfinished business from the previous phase can complicate or block movement through the transitions. Families or individuals can become permanently frozen in an adaptive structure that has outlived its utility (Penn, 1983). For example, the usefulness of pulling together in the crisis period can become a maladaptive and stifling prison for all family members in the chronic phase. Enmeshed families, because of their rigid and fused nature, would have difficulty negotiating this delicate transition. A family that is adept at handling the day-to-day practicalities of a long-term stable illness but limited in its skills in affective coping may encounter difficulty if its family member's disease becomes terminal. The relatively greater demand for affective coping skills in the terminal versus the chronic phase of an illness may create a crisis for a family navigating this transition.

The time phases and typology of illness provide a framework for a chronic disease psychosocial developmental model. The time phases (crisis, chronic, and terminal) can be considered broad developmental periods in the natural history of chronic disease. Each period has certain basic tasks independent of the type of illness. In addition to the phase-specific developmental tasks common to all psychosocial types of disease, each "type" of illness has specific supplementary tasks. This is analogous to the relationship between a particular individual's development and certain universal life tasks. The basic tasks of the three illness time phases and transitions recapitulate in many respects the unfolding of human development. For example, the crisis phase is similar in certain fundamental ways to the era of childhood and adolescence. Normal child development involves a prolonged period of learning to assimilate from and accommodate to the fundamentals of life. Parents often temper other developmental plans (e.g., career) to accommodate raising children. Likewise, the crisis phase is a period of socialization to the basics of living with chronic disease. During this phase, other life pans are frequently put on hold by the family to accommodate the socialization to illness process. Themes of separation and individuation are central in the transition from adolescence to adulthood. One must relinquish a moratorium in terms of assuming normal adult responsibilities. In a similar way, the transition to the chronic phase of illness emphasizes autonomy and the creation of a viable ongoing life structure given the realities of the illness (life). In the transition to the chronic phase a "hold" or moratorium on other developmental tasks that served to protect the initial period of socialization/adaptation to life with chronic disease is reevaluated.

At this point, we can combine the typology and phases of illness to construct a two dimensional matrix (see Figure 4). This matrix permits the grouping and differentiation of illnesses according to important similarities or differences. It subdivides types of chronic illnesses into three time phases. This allows examination of a chronic illness in a more refined way.

By the addition of a family systems model to this matrix, we can create a three dimensional representation of the broader illness/family system (see Figure 5). Psychosocial illness types, time phases of illness, and components of family functioning constitute the three dimensions. This model offers a vehicle for flexible dialogue between the illness aspect and family aspect of the illness/family system. In essence, this model allows speculation about the importance of strengths and weaknesses in various components of family functioning in relation to different types of disease at different phases in the illness life cycle.

CLINICAL IMPLICATIONS

There are several important implications of this model for clinical practice. At their core, the components of the typology provide a means to grasp the character of a chronic illness in psychosocial terms. They provide a meaningful bridge for the clinician between the biological and psychosocial worlds. Perhaps the major contribution is the provision of a framework for assessment and clinical intervention with a family facing a chronic or life-threatening illness. The clinician can think with greater clarity and focus. Attention to features of onset, course, outcome, and incapacitation provide markers that facilitate integration of an assessment. This will focus a clinician's questioning of a family. For instance, acute onset illnesses demand high levels of adaptability, problem solving, role reallocation, and balanced cohesion. A high degree of family enmeshment, might make a family less likely to be able to cope with these demands. Forethought on this issue would cue a clinician toward a more appropriate family evaluation.

The concept of time phases provides a way for the clinician to think longitudinally, and to reach a fuller understanding of chronic illness as an ongoing process with landmarks, transition points, and changing demands. An illness time line delineates psychosocial developmental stages of an illness, each phase with its own unique developmental tasks. Kaplan (1968) has emphasized the importance of solving phase related tasks within the time limits set by the duration of each successive developmental phase of an illness. He suggests the failure to re-

ONSET	COURSE	OUTCOME	INCAPACITATION
A = acute	P = progressive	F = fatal or shortened	Yes = (+)
G = gradual	C = constant	lifespan	No = (–)
	R = relapsing	NF = nonfatal	

	I CRISIS	PHASE II CHRONIC	III TERMINAL
A P F +			
A P F –			
A P NF +			
A P NF –			
A C F +			
A C F –			
A C NF +			
A C NF –			
A R F +			
A R F –			
A R NF +			
A R NF +			
ILLNESS TYPE			
G P F +			
G P F –			
G P NF +			
G P NF –			
G C F +			
G C F –			
G C NF +			
G C NF –			
G R F +			
G R F –			
G R NF +			
G R NF –			

FIGURE 4. Matrix of Illness Types and Time Phases. Reprinted by permission from *Family Systems Medicine*, 2:3, pp. 245-262.

solve issues in this sequential manner can jeopardize the total coping process of the family. Therefore, attention to time allows the clinician to assess a family's strengths and vulnerabilities in relation to the present and future phases of the illness.

Taken together the typology and time phases provide a context to integrate other aspects of a comprehensive assessment. This would involve evaluation of a range of universal and illness specific family dynamics in relation to the psychosocial type and time phases of illness. This could include assessment of: the family's illness belief system; the meaning of the illness to the family; the interface of the illness with individual and family development; the family's transgenerational history of coping with illness, loss, and crisis; the family's medical crisis planning; the family's capacity to perform home-based medical care; and the family's illness-oriented communication, problem solving, role reallocation, affective involvement, social support, and use of community resources.

An example can highlight the interplay of the psychosocial type of illness with future developmental transitions. Imagine a family in which the father, a carpenter and primary financial provider, develops multiple sclerosis. At first, his level of impairment is mild and stabilized. This allows him to continue part-time work. Because their children are all teenagers, his wife is able to undertake part-time work to help maintain financial stability. The oldest son, age 15, seems rela-

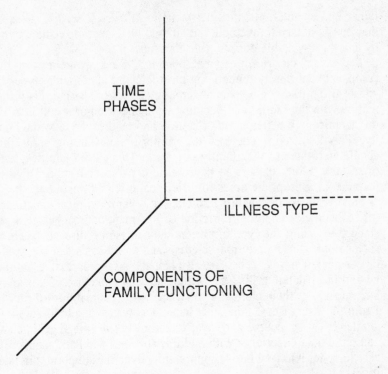

FIGURE 5. Three Dimensional Model: Illness Type, Time Phase, Family Functioning.

tively unaffected. Two years later, father experiences a rapid progression of his illness leaving him totally disabled. His son, now 17, has dreams of going away to college and getting educated for a career in science. The specter of financial hardship and the perceived need for a "man in the family" creates a serious dilemma of choice for the son and the family. In this case there is a fundamental clash between developmental issues of separation/individuation and the ongoing demands of progressive chronic disability upon the family. This vignette demonstrates the potential clash between simultaneous transition periods: the illness transition to a more incapacitating and progressive course, the adolescent son's transition to early adulthood, and the family's transition from the "living with teenagers" to "launching young adults" stage. Also, this example illustrates the significance of the type of illness. An illness that was less incapacitating or relapsing (as opposed to a progressive or constant course disease) might interfere less with this young man's separation from his family of origin. If his father had an intermittently incapacitating illness, like disc disease, the son might have moved out but tailored his choices to remain close by and thus available during acute flare-ups.

The model clarifies treatment planning. First, awareness of the components of family functioning most relevant to particular types or phases of an illness guides goal-setting. The act of sharing this information with the family and deciding upon specific goals will provide therapeutically a better sense of control and realistic hope to the family. This knowledge educates the family about warning signs that should alert them to seek family treatment. This guides families, who often lack prior exposure to psychiatric care, to call upon a family therapist at appropriate times for brief goal-oriented treatment.

Finally, the model enables clinicians to organize clinical experience for realistic extension or restriction of treatment approaches. For instance, by using the typology seemingly disparate diseases such as rheumatoid arthritis, multiple sclerosis and Parkinson's disease would be considered similar. They are all gradual onset, progressive, nonfatal and incapacitating illnesses. Clinicians can make use of this similarity to apply their clinical experience with rheumatoid arthritis to Parkinson's disease. On the other hand, a slow growing brain tumor is similar in onset, course and incapacitation, but it is fatal. Clinicians could use their experience with multiple sclerosis and Parkinson's disease but alter it to take into account family dynamics important in fatal illness.

RESEARCH IMPLICATIONS

The model has important implications for research. First, reexamination of previous studies using this model might clarify some of the confusion surrounding conflicting results or lack of statistical significance. Stratification by illness type and/or time phase might bring significant associations to light.

Cognizance of the time phases is essential to study design. It is crucial that an investigator is aware of which time phase — crisis, chronic or terminal — a case is in as it enters a study for assessment or intervention. Different results are quite likely if studies differ in their timing. The time phases can clarify a methodology for longitudinal studies. Multiple observations could be spaced at intervals that correspond to the different time periods.

The typology should facilitate research designed to sort out the relative importance of different psychosocial variables across a spectrum of diseases. Grouping illnesses by the parameters of this typology should help in this regard. According to the premises for this typology, illnesses appearing within the same category have qualitatively and quantitatively the highest congruence of psychosocial demands on the family. In other words, pooling results from studies of Parkinson's disease, rheumatoid arthritis, chronic obstructive pulmonary diseases and multiple sclerosis (all gradual onset/progressive course/incapacitating/nonfatal) would allow significant generalizations for that cluster of diseases. Illnesses within a particular category can be considered crudely matched as to type of onset, course, outcome and incapacitation. Since each of these variables exists as a continuum, the degree of homogeneity of study cases can be fine-tuned according to the desire of the investigator. Specific criteria for subdivisions are feasible for any of the typology's variables.

Theoretically, the typology enables us to more easily isolate a "critical" aspect of chronic illness for more intensive study. For instance, one might ask, "What is the relative importance of family adaptability for chronic diseases with and without incapacitation?" A comparison could be made between two types of illnesses that vary with respect to the presence or absence of incapacitation but are matched for the other typology attributes. So, lumbo-sacral disc disease (*Incapacitating/acute onset/relapsing/nonfatal*) and peptic ulcer disease (*Non-incapacitating/acute* or gradual onset/relapsing/nonfatal) could be used to investigate the relative importance of high versus low family adaptability in incapacitating versus non-incapacitating diseases.

Also, the model simplifies the design of studies intended to explore the interactional effects of the components of the typology. As an extension of the hypothetical study just described, by using a 2 × 2 design one could investigate how fatal versus nonfatal outcome interacts with the presence or absence of incapacitation.

Overall, the typology and time phase matrix provides a framework to generate and test hypotheses about the relationship of different components of family or individual functioning to disease course for different types and phases of illness. Referring back to Figure 5, if we operationalize the typology, time phases of illness and components of family functioning as three distinct variables then three kinds of prototypical comparisons can be generated by holding any two variables constant. This would allow asking the following sorts of questions: (1) given illness type X in the crisis phase, how does high versus low family cohesion affect disease course; (2) given illness type X with high family cohesion, how is disease course affected in each of the three time phases; (3) how does high family cohesion in the chronic phase affect the course of different types of illnesses?

The implications to research can be summarized. Use of the model for reanalysis of previous studies may lead to new insights. The model will significantly improve our ability to generate more succinct hypotheses. Definitions of independent and dependent variables will be clearer. Components of the typology and time phases of illness clarify what to control in a study design. Used in conjunction with a well-researched family systems model like the McMaster (Epstein et al., 1978; Epstein & Bishop, 1981; Epstein et al., 1984), Structural (Minuchin et al., 1978; Minuchin et al., 1975), Beavers-Timberlawn (Lewis et al., 1977) or Circumplex (Olson et al., 1979, 1979; Olson & McCubbin, 1981; Russell, 1979; Sprenkle & Olson, 1978), the typology should improve family systems medicine research.

CLINICAL APPLICATIONS: THE THERAPEUTIC QUADRANGLE

Using the psychosocial typology and time phases of illness as a reference point has important implications for health services delivery both for the patient/family's relationship to health professionals and for the organization of services.

Haley (1976) observed that helping professionals need to be included in the conceptualization of any therapeutic treatment system with a family. The application of this idea in the medical world has led to various descriptions of "the Therapeutic Triangle in Medicine" (Doherty & Baird 1983). This triangle includes the patient, his/her family, and the physician (health care team). Doherty and Baird point out the illusory nature of thinking in dyadic terms about the patient-family and physician-patient relationships. They stress active participation of the physician in the former and the family in the latter. A schematic representation of this set of relationships looks like that depicted in Figure 6.

The inclusion of the concept of psychosocial illness "types" into the scheme creates a four member system composed of four interlocking triangles (see Figure 7). It is easier to conceptualize the illness as a fourth member if one pictures each illness "type" as having a personality (which includes the kind of onset, course, outcome, degree of incapacitation, and predictability) and developmental life course (which includes the time phases of chronic illness).

Within this paradigm, one might take the original therapeutic triangle diagrammed in Figure 6 (the patient, the family, and the health care team) and see how it is colored by different types of illness. For instance, consider the concept of locus of control in relation to disease

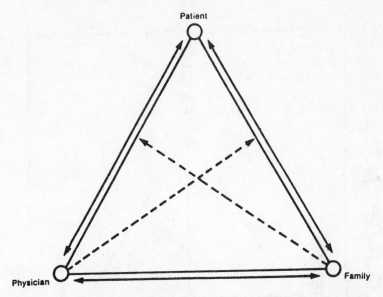

FIGURE 6. The Therapeutic Triangle in Medicine. Excerpted from *Family Therapy and Family Medicine: Toward the Primary Care of Families*, by W. J. Doherty and M. A. Baird. 1983. New York: The Guilford Press. Reprinted by permission.

(Wallston et al., 1976, 1978). A family's beliefs about the potential to control biological processes can vary along a continuum from an internal to external orientation. A certain minimal level of agreement concerning this kind of health belief is critical for the establishment of a viable therapeutic relationship between the patient, his/her family, and the health care team. The degree of consensus concerning locus of control can vary dramatically for this triad depending on the "type" of chronic disease. A particular family physician may have had a good working relationship with a family that had presented over the years with non-life-threatening and non-incapacitating illnesses. If the father suffers a serious heart attack and there are differences in beliefs about control which surface in relation to this more life-threatening and incapacitating illness, the stability of the longstanding therapeutic triangle might be threatened. If the physician checked his/her own beliefs and questioned the family about theirs in relation to a life-threatening incapacitating disease, a potential serious rift in this therapeutic system might be averted.

The therapeutic quadrangle also allows analysis of how a particular

THE THERAPEUTIC QUADRANGLE

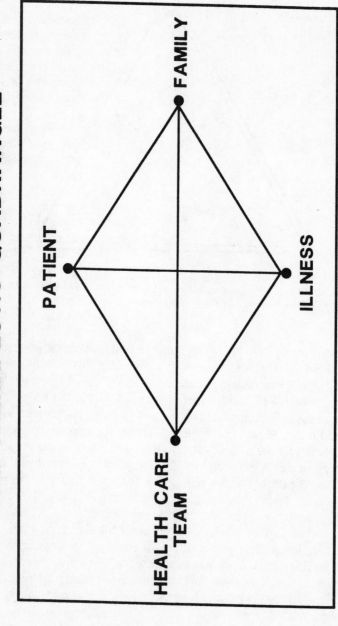

FIGURE 7

164

psychosocial type of illness interfaces with the health care team's relationship with the family and the patient independently.

In terms of the organization of services, the psychosocial typology and time phases of illness have implications for periodic reevaluation of the family in relation to the illness life cycle. The time phases and transition points suggest the timing of the evaluations. Strengths and weaknesses in various components of family functioning can thus be addressed taking into account all relevant factors related to the "psychosocial type" of the illness.

The typology facilitates the development of various patient support or psycho-educational groups for families. For example, groups could be designed to meet the needs of patients dealing with: progressive, life-threatening diseases; relapsing disorders; acute onset, incapacitating illnesses; or the chronic phase of constant course diseases. Sometimes there are not enough families involved with any particular disease to form such groups. This is particularly relevant in more rural settings or for less common illnesses. Thinking about group-oriented services in terms of illness types helps to overcome these obstacles while maintaining the groups' thematic coherence. Also, packaging brief psycho-educational "modules" timed for critical phases of particular "types" of diseases, encourages families to accept and digest manageable portions of a long-term coping process. Each module could be tailored to the particular phase of the illness life cycle and family coping skills necessary to confront disease-related demands. This would provide a cost-effective preventive service that could also aid in the detection of families at high risk for maladaptation to chronic illness.

CONCLUSION

The purpose of this paper has been to describe a conceptual model that clarifies thinking about the system created at the interface of chronic illness with the family. Several problems were identified as major impediments to progress in this field. These difficulties suggested the need for: (1) a categorization scheme that organizes similarities and differences between diseases in a manner useful to psychosocial rather than medical inquiry; and (2) greater attention to the variation of illnesses over their time course.

A three-dimensional model emerges in the process of addressing these needs. On the first dimension, psychosocial "types" of illnesses are created based on combinations of four components: onset, course, outcome, and degree of incapacitation. The second dimension distinguishes three phases in the life history of chronic disease: crisis, chronic, and terminal. The third dimension includes various universal and illness specific components of family functioning. A more detailed discussion of this third dimension and in particular disease-oriented family dynamics appears in a separate paper (Rolland, in press). This model provides a way to better appreciate the illness/family system. It does this by facilitating interactional thinking about the relationships between the illness type, the time phases of illness, and family functioning.

As a cornerstone of this three-dimensional model, the typology of illness can facilitate a key goal of family systems medicine to integrate a number of sovereign territories into a truly coherent discipline (Bloch, 1983). When used in an interlocking way with typological models of the family or an illness-oriented family assessment, this categorization scheme provides the researcher and clinician with a clearer path into this rich forest. In clinical practice, it will be most helpful when applied in the initial diagnostic phase of the illness, when the family and health care providers must come to grips with the myriad of issues surrounding medical treatment and family system coping and adaptation.

REFERENCES

Adams, J.E. & Lindemann, E. (1974). Coping with long-term disability. In Coelho, G.V., Hamburg, D.A. & Adams, J.E. (Eds.) *Coping and Adaptation*. New York: Basic Books, Inc.

Atcherberg, J., Lawlis, G.F., Simonton, O.C. & Mathews-Simonton, S. (1977). Psychological factors and blood chemistries as disease outcome predictors for cancer patients. *Multivariate Exp Clin Research, 3*, 107-122.

Baker, L., Minuchin, S., Milman, L. et al. (1975). Psychosomatic aspects of juvenile diabetes mellitus: A progress report. *In Modern Problems in Pediatrics, 12*, White Plains, NY: S. Karger.

Bishop, D.S. & Epstein, N.B. (1980). Family problems and disability. In Bishop, D.S. (Ed.), *Behavior Problems and the Disabled: Assessment and Management*. Baltimore, MD: Williams and Wilkins.

Bishop, D.S., Epstein, N.B. & Baldwin, L.M. (1982). Disability: A family affair. In Freeman, D.S. & Trute, B. (Eds.). *Treating Families with Special Needs*. Alberta Assoc of Social Workers and Canadian Assoc of Social Workers.

Bloch, D.A. (1983). Family systems medicine: The field and the journal. *Family Systems Medicine, 1*, No. 1, 3-12.

Blumberg, E.M., West, P.H. & Ellis, F.W. (1954). A possible relationship between psychological factors and human cancer. *Psychosomatic Medicine, 16*, 277-286.

Bradley, C. (1979). Life events and the control of diabetes mellitus. *Journal of Psychosomatic Research, 23*, 159-162.

Carter, E.A. & McGoldrick M. (Eds.). (1980). *The Family Life Cycle: A Framework for Family Therapy*. New York: Gardner Press.

Chodoff, P., Friedman, S.B. & Hamburg, D.A. (1964). Stress, defenses and coping behavior: Observations in parents of children with malignant disease. *American Journal of Psychiatry, 120*, 743-749.

Cleveland, M. (1980). Family adaptation to traumatic spinal cord injury, response to crisis. *Family Relations, 29*, 558-565.

Croog, S.H., Shapiro, D.S. & Levine, S. (1971). Denial among male heart patients: An empirical study. *Psychosomatic Medicine, 33*, 385-397.

Davies, R.K., Quinlan, D.M., McKegney, P. & Kimball, C.P. (1973). Organic factors and psychological adjustment in advanced cancer patients. *Psychosomatic Medicine, 35*, 464-471.

Derogatis, L.R., Abeloff, M.D. & Melisartos, N. (1979). Psychological coping mechanisms and survival time in metastatic breast cancer. *Journal of the American Medical Association, 242*, 1504-1508.

Doherty, W.J. & Baird, M.A. (1983). *Family Therapy and Family Medicine: Toward the Primary Care of Families*. New York: Guilford Press.

Elliott, G.R. & Eisdorfer, C. (1982). *Stress and Human Health: Analysis and Implications of Research*. New York: Springer.

Engel, G.H. (1977). The need for a new medical model: A challenge for biomedicine. *Science, 196*, 129-136.

Engel, G.H. (1980). The clinical application of the biopsychosocial model. *American Journal of Psychiatry, 137*, 535-544.

Epstein, N.B., Bishop, D.S. & Levin, S. (1978). McMaster model of family functioning. *J Marriage and Family Counselling, 4*, 19-31.

Epstein, N.B. & Bishop, D.S. (1981). Problem-centered systems therapy of the family. In Gurman, A. and Kniskern, D. (Eds.), *Handbook of Family Therapy*. New York: Brunner/Mazel.

Epstein, N.B., Baldwin, L.M. & Bishop, D.S. (1983). The McMaster family assessment device. *Amer J of Family Therapy*.

Fox, B.H. (1982). A psychological measure as a predictor in cancer. In Cohen, J., Cullen, W. & Martin, L.R. (Eds.), *Psychological Aspects of Cancer*. New York: Raven Press.

Hackett, T.P., Cassem, N.H. & Wishnie, H.A. (1968). The coronary-care unit: An appraisal of its psychologic hazards. *New England Journal of Medicine, 279*, 1365-1370.

Haley, J. (1976). *Problem Solving Therapy*. San Francisco: Jossey-Bass.

Hamburg, B.A., Lipsett, L.F., Inoff, G.E. & Drash, A.L. (Eds.). (1980). *Behavioral and Psychological Issues in Diabetes*. U.S. Government Printing Office, NIH Publication No. 80-1993.

Hyman, M. (1975). Social and psychological factors affecting disability among ambulatory patients. *J of Chronic Diseases, 28*, 199-216.

Kaplan, D.M. (1968). Observations on crisis theory and practice. *Social Casework, 49*, 151-155.

Kasl, S.V. (1982). Social and psychological factors affecting the course of disease: an epidemiological perspective. In Mechanic, D. (Ed.), *Handbook of Health, Health Care and the Health Profession*. New York: Free Press.

Levinson, D.J. (1978). *The Seasons of a Man's Life*. New York: Knopf.

Lewis, J.H., Beavers, W.R., Gossett, J.T. & Phillips, V.A. (1977). *No Single Thread: Psychological Health in Family Systems*. New York: Brunner/Mazel.

Litman, T.J. (1974). The family as a basic unit in health and medical care: A social behavioral overview. *Social Science and Medicine, 8*, 495-519.

Matus, I. & Bush, D. (1979). Asthma attack frequency in a pediatric population. *Psychosomatic Medicine, 41*, 629-636.

Minuchin, S., Rosman, B.L. & Baker, L. (1978). *Psychosomatic Families*. Cambridge, MA: Harvard University Press.

Minuchin, S., Baker, L., Rosman, B., Liebman, R., Milman, L. & Todd, T. (1975). A conceptual model of psychosomatic illness in children: Family organization and family therapy. *Archives of General Psychiatry, 32*, 1031-1038.

Moldofsky, H. & Chester, W.J. (1970). Pain and mood patterns in patients with rheumatoid arthritis: A prospective study. *Psychosomatic Medicine, 32*, 309-318.

Moos, R.H. (Ed.). (1984). *Coping with Physical Illness, 2: New Perspectives*. New York: Plenum Publishing.

Olson, D., Sprenkle, D.H. & Russell, C.S. (1979). Circumplex model of marital and family systems I: Cohesion and adaptability dimensions, family types, and clinical applications. *Family Process, 18*, 3-28.

Olson, D.H., Russell, C.S. & Sprenkle, D.H. (1979). Circumplex model of marital family systems II: Empirical studies and clinical intervention. In Vincent, J. (Ed.), *Advances in Family Intervention, Assessment and Theory*. Greenwich, CN: JAI Press, 128-176.

Olson, D.H. & McCubbin, H.I. (1981). Circumplex model of marital and family systems V: Application to family stress and crisis intervention. In McCubbin, H.I. (Ed.), *Family Stress, Coping, and Social Support*. New York: Springer Publishing.

Penn, P. (1983). Coalitions and binding interactions in families with chronic illness. *Family Systems Medicine, 1*(2), 16-25.

Rolland, J.S. (1984). Toward a psychosocial typology of chronic and life-threatening illness. *Family Systems Medicine, 2*(3), 245-263.

Rolland, J.S. (in press). Family systems and chronic illness: A conceptual model. In Dym, B., & Berman, S. (Eds.). New York: Brunner/Mazel.

Rolland, J.S. (1987). Chronic illnes and the life cycle: A conceptual framework. *Family Process, 26*, 203-221.

Russell, C.S. (1979). Circumplex model of marital and family systems III; Empirical evaluation with families. *Family Process, 18*, 29-45.

Schmale, A.H. & Iker, H. (1971). Hopelessness as a predictor of cervical cancer. *Soc Sci Med. 5*, 95-100.

Simonton, C.O., Mathews-Simonton, S. & Sparks, T.F. (1980). Psychological intervention in the treatment of cancer. *Psychosomatics, 21*(3), 226-233.

Slater, S.B., Sussman, M.B. & Stroud, M.W. (1970). Participation in household activities as a prognostic factor for rehabilitation. *Archives of Physical Medicine and Rehabilitation, 51*, 605-611.

Sourkes, B.M. (1982). *The Deepening Shade: Psychological Aspects of Long-term Illness*. Pittsburgh: University of Pittsburgh Press.

Sprenkle, D.H. & Olson, D.H. (1978). Circumplex model of marital and family systems IV: Empirical study of clinic and non-clinic couples. *Journal of Marital and Family Therapy, 4*, 59-74.

Sussman, M.B. & Slater, S.B. (1971). Reappraisal of urban kin networks: Empirical evidence. *The Annals, 396*, 40.

Swanson, D.W. & Maruta, J. (1980). The family's viewpoint of chronic pain. *Pain, 8*, 163-166.

Turk, J. (1964). Impact of cystic fibrosis on family functioning. *Pediatrics, 34*, 67-71.

Viney, L.L. & Westbrook, M.T. (1981). Psychosocial reactions to chronic illness related disability as a function of its severity and type. *Journal of Psychosomatic Research, 25*, (6), 513-523.

Wallston, B.S., Wallston, K.A., Kaplan, G.D. & Maides, S.A. (1976). Development and validation of the Health Locus of Control (HLC) Scale. *Journal of Consulting and Clinical Psychology, 44*, 580-585.

Wallston, K.A. & Wallston, B.S. (1978). Development of the Multidimensional Health Locus of Control (MHLC) Scales. *Health Education Monographs, Vol 6*, No. 2, 160-170.

Weiss, H.M. (1983). Personal Communication.

Weiss, S.M., Herd, J.A. & Fox, B.H. (Eds.). (1981). *Perspectives on Behavioral Medicine*. New York: Academic Press.

Wolff, C.T., Friedman, S.B., Hofer, M.A. & Mason, J.W. (1964). Relationship between psychological defenses and mean urinary 17-hydroxy corticosteriod excretion rate. I. A predictive study of parents of fatally ill children. *Psychosomatic Medicine, 26*, 576-591.

The Family System
and the Health Care System:
Making the Invisible Visible

Evan Imber-Black

INTRODUCTION

Case Vignette #1

A family consisting of a mother and father, Mr. and Mrs. B., in their late 50s and a 22-year-old son, Robert, were referred for a consultation. The son had been diabetic since childhood, and was presently functioning poorly in all aspects of life. In addition to his diabetes, he often had severe angry outbursts which frightened his mother and from which his father distanced. He lived at home with his parents, who were in severe conflict regarding his present care and his future. Since he had had many life threatening insulin reactions and diabetic comas, the mother wanted to keep him at home and look after him, while the father believed that the son needed more independence. At the consultation, several professionals involved with the young man and his family were also present. Robert's primary physician strongly believed Robert should leave home and live in an extended care hospital. He believed no efforts should be made towards independent living, citing both Robert's brittle diabetes and his behavior problems. A social worker, with the social service department which paid Robert an income every month, believed Robert should try to live on his own, and begin to work. A specialist who saw Robert and his mother during crises strongly believed Robert should remain at home. During the interview, it became apparent that conflicting views regarding Robert, his care and his prognosis had existed for several years, across many issues, and involving *many* professionals in addition to the ones present in the interview. Family members, especially

Evan Imber-Black, Director of Family and Group Studies, and Associate Professor, Department of Psychiatry, Albert Einstein College of Medicine, Bronx, NY.

Mrs. B., expressed deep worry and anxiety about choosing the advice of one helper over another, and recounted incidents in which she felt quite paralyzed lest she make the wrong decision and lose the support of the professionals involved with her son.

Case Vignette #2

A couple, Mr. and Mrs. Leon, in their mid-30s, were referred for a consultation. The couple had three young children. Mr. Leon had chronic migraine headaches since young adulthood. He had coped with the headaches until two years ago when they worsened, and he began several stays in the hospital. Recently, he lost his job, and Mrs. Leon began to work outside the home for a minimum wage. The consultation was requested by the hospital because all medical efforts were failing, a psychiatric hypothesis was being considered, since Mr. Leon was extremely depressed, *and* because hospital personnel were in great conflict with Mrs. Leon. What emerged during the interview were the disparate beliefs that Mr. and Mrs. Leon held towards traditional health care. Mr. Leon stated that he had *absolute* faith in modern medicine, and that he was certain that in time the hospital would help him. Mrs. Leon believed in holistic healing, and felt betrayed by what she saw as her husband's alliance with medical personnel, who, in fact, were not helping him. She felt he was a "guinea pig," and was extremely angry with him for allowing this, and with the hospital for continuing to treat him, despite repeated failures. She recounted several angry interactions between herself and hospital personnel that she believed were the result of her refusal to agree with their treatment plans. Over time, her husband's physicians told her less and less regarding their decisions. Mr. Leon stated that he felt extremely caught between his wife's views and those of his doctors, and that no matter which way he turned, he would be the "loser."

Case Vignette #3

A family consisting of a single parent, Mrs. Dobbs, her 13- year-old daughter, Kelly, and seven-year-old son, John, were referred for family therapy. Kelly had developed what she identified as severe upper abdominal pains one year earlier. A lengthy period of diagnosis and multiple hospital stays ensued. Each attempt to discern Kelly's problem was unsuccessful. Due to such lack of success, professionals speculated that Kelly's problems were psychosomatic, and reports were written that blamed Kelly's family. Most recently, from further tests, Kelly had been given a biomedical diagnosis.

Mrs. Dobbs was the sole support of the family. Kelly's father had left the family five years earlier, sent no money, and did not visit Kelly. Hospital personnel were extremely critical of Mrs. Dobbs because she did not visit Kelly "enough." Mrs. Dobbs worked full-time at a low paying job, and had no one who could watch John in the evenings, except paid babysitters. At the same time, since Mrs. Dobbs asked many questions and expressed frustration at the lack of progress, she was designated as "overinvolved," resulting in the referral for family therapy, which Mrs. Dobbs did not understand. During the interview, Mrs. Dobbs also recounted a history with other larger systems, including the school system, and public welfare, in which she felt judged critically for being a poor, single parent, without formal education and from which she felt mystified and not given adequate information.

PROBLEMATIC ISSUES, PATTERNS AND THEMES

All of these vignettes, and many more like them in which families have ill or disabled members (including physical illness, psychiatric problems, and mental handicaps), share a common and crucial dimension that is seldom examined, namely that such families are *required* to interact with multiple helpers and larger systems. In turn, the larger systems, who generally define their work as being on behalf of an individual patient, in fact, are *required* to interact with families. This salient feature, that families with an ill or handicapped member and the larger systems providing services are uniquely involved with one another, is often ignored or otherwise made invisible. When attended to, each family/larger system interaction is viewed as "special," reflecting the idiosyncracies of one particular family member, and, perhaps, one or two individual helpers (for instance "that husband and that nurse do not get along" or "Mrs. Z makes trouble when she visits her son," etc.).

In fact, the relationships between families with ill or handicapped members and the larger systems can be profitably examined and assessed for commonalities across cases that impact on family functioning and on larger system functioning in their shared member's behalf. Here, our familiar skills in assessing family patterns may be shifted to the more inclusive level of family and larger system. Features of an assessment model to examine family/larger system relationships include:

1. Dyadic Patterns

The first element of assessment is dyadic patterns. The family system and the health care system also may usefully be examined as a dyadic relationship in which the participants are either seeking and attempting to define a *complementary* relationship, marked by an exchange of different behaviors that fit and imply one another, such as care giver and care receiver, or a *symmetrical* relationship, marked by an exchange of similar behaviors and partnership.

The health care system generally defines its relationship to families and to patients as complementary. Thus, there is a rigid definition of care provider and care receiver, of decisionmaker and recipient of decisions. Occasionally a more symmetrical partnership or collaboration is invoked. When families, either directly or implicitly challenge this definition, conflict often ensues.

Dyadic struggles between family member and health care providers frequently emerge over definitions of the problem to be addressed and the preferred solutions. (Thus, in the vignette cited earlier, Mrs. Leon's very different ideas about health care were seen as "kooky" and were ignored. In turn, Mrs. Leon became more adamant in her refusal to support medical efforts in her husband's behalf, and a ferocious escalation ensued in which the health care system implemented more and more invasive procedures, with no progress, while Mrs. Leon became more and more angry with hospital personnel *and* with her husband for permitting the procedures.) Here, the refusal on the part of a family member to accept a complementary relationship, and the refusal by the health care system to entertain alternative relationship options, resulted in deterioration of the patient, the couple and the family-larger system relationship. Neither a workable complementarity, nor a viable symmetry prevailed, but rather a symmetrical escalation took hold over "who knew best."

A second problem may emerge when the complementary nature of the relationship escalates such that the patient and/or family members become more and more helpless in the face of more and more help. (In the same example, as Mrs. Leon and the hospital became embroiled in symmetrical conflict, the relationship of Mr. Leon and the hospital was marked by escalating complementarity, as he became more and more needy and the hospital tried more and more efforts that failed.) An adolescent boy poignantly described this dyadic pattern to me in an interview when he said of his single parent mother "all of the help she needs for my retarded sister makes her feel helpless, as she becomes more and more helpless, they give her more and more help."

2. Triadic Patterns

The second element of assessment is triadic patterns. Moving from a focus on a unit of two to a unit of three, issues of organization and power in interacting systems emerge. Family therapists have, of course, long looked at triads *within* the family.

Moving to a more inclusive level, one can see that family members and health care providers easily create *inadvertent* triads that handicap functioning for all concerned. The family system and the larger system often hold emotional and physical survival value for an ill person. Thus, when these systems or members within these systems are in conflict, the patient is caught in a triangle of *special proportions*. Sometimes, such triangles may mirror already existing family process, as in the vignette of the diabetic boy, his family and helpers (Imber-Coppersmith, 1983, 1985; Schwartzman, 1985). Here, splits in the family regarding the patient are *replicated* by splits among the helpers, creating a complex and reified macrosystem. In this situation, it is not unusual to see a process marked by the continual search for allies, as family members and helpers seek out others to be "on their side."

It is important to note, however, that triangles in the macrosystem may not necessarily indicate intra-family triangles, but may simply be the result of two *very* different systems, the informal family and the formal and bureaucratic health care system, encountering each other. Often, triangles in the system formed by family and health care system are unnoticed, and, rather, interactions marked by individual blame, criticism and mistrust are given attention. Further, such triangles may be exacerbated by the entry of related systems, such as welfare, schools, group homes or therapy.

3. Boundaries

The third element of assessment is boundaries. When a family has a severely or chronically ill member, the boundaries of the family must shift, sometimes profoundly, in order to accommodate the entry of the health care system. It is important to note that it is the family's boundaries which are required to undergo change in order to accommodate the health care system, and not vice versa. Families who do not like or do not understand the working of a health care system generally have little choice in the matter. For instance, families must follow hospital regulations, or be "invited" to leave. When the illness or handicap is long-lasting, the family's boundary organization vis-à-vis outside systems must, likewise, undergo long-lasting change.

Here the family's history with larger systems may be salient. Thus, a family that has been private, isolated or otherwise disengaged from large, formal systems, may have an especially difficult time. Distancing from the larger systems' entry may be easily misunderstood as lack of interest in their ill member, rather than an initial inability to alter boundaries. If the health care system distances in turn as often happens then a macrosystem marked by rigid, impermeable boundaries may develop.

Conversely, one or more family members may become enmeshed with representatives of the larger system. Here, one sees a pattern in which members of the health care system become involved in family issues that are well beyond the purview of appropriate patient care; such enmeshment may deleteriously effect intra-family relationships, as, for instance, when a mother confides more and more in her child's nurse, and less and less in her husband.

When a family "designates" one member to interact with the larger system, the likelihood of boundary problems, both within the family and between the family and the health care system increases. For its part the health care system often contributes to this problem when, reflecting wider cultural norms, appointments are set to include mothers and not fathers. In this conduit position, frequently supported by family and health care system alike, mothers may then experience the doublebinding message that they are "overinvolved."

The boundaries between the family system and the health care system may exhibit an unusual combination of diffusion and rigidity. Information about the family's life may be readily exchanged in the health care system, while information from the health care system regarding plans, policy changes, etc., may not be shared with the family. The "door" to the family system may be required to be opened to multiple health care providers, while the "door" to the health care system is highly regulated by formal processes.

4. Myths and Beliefs

The fourth element of assessment is myths and beliefs. The family system and the larger systems seldom share enough information with each other, leading to misunderstanding and confusion. It is as if representatives of these systems speak to each other with large synapses. Thus, a family's circumstances are often not understood and inappropriate judgements are made and acted upon. Families' particular ways of imparting and processing information may be ignored. The working processes of the larger systems are often not explained to families, who, rather, are expected to simply "fit in." Often, the reasons for decisions, the rationale for referrals, changing policies, etc., are not given to family members and many families lack the skills to inquire, including knowing what questions to ask or whom to ask. A sense of helplessness may then translate into anger, leading to further distancing by the health care system. Lacking specific information, both families and larger systems are forced to fill in what's missing with their own, often mistaken fantasies, which, when acted upon, may lead to further misunderstanding.

Families with severely or chronically ill members have often developed fixed beliefs or myths about the health care system, or specific categories of health care providers (for instance, nurses, doctors, specialists, social workers, etc.). Very often, critical incidents occurring between the family and health care system serve to shape such myths. Such critical incidents may often occur at points of diagnoses or at key transition points in a patient's care, when both family and providers are anxious. In turn, health care personnel develop myths regarding certain health conditions and particular families. For instance, a common myth among workers with the mentally handicapped is that their families are also intellectually deficient (Sarason & Doris, 1979). Such myths may generate modes of interaction that are repetitive, stereotypic and myth-supporting.

5. Multiple Embedded Systems

The fifth element of assessment is an examination of multiple embedded systems. It is the tradition of *most* health care systems to view problems in isolation, and while causal hypotheses linking a problem to a family context may be offered, these are generally unidirectional and blame oriented, rather than interactive at either the family *or* especially the family-larger systems level. The complex embedded system of patient-family-health care providers/community-social norms and values is seldom seen as a locus for assessment and intervention. Rather, an individualistic view prevails, not capable of understanding the multiple helper system that begins to emerge with characteristics of its own. Rather than conceptualizing the problem as a family-multiple helper system, the locus of blame is placed *in* the family with the designation "multiple-problem" family. Further, social norms, values, and circumstances that profoundly shape the service delivery system remain hidden, including sexism, racism, classism, ageism, and attitudes towards particular human conditions (such as the mentally handicapped). Thus, in the vignette discussed earlier the *attitudes* towards Kelly's mother as a poor, female, single parent were *never* examined by the providers as part of the salient system.

I'd like to turn now to a longer case example which illustrates the issues. I've called this case "The Potato and the Kiwi Fruit" for reasons which will become obvious (see Figure 1).

A family was referred by a dietician due to the "severe eating disorder" of Sandra, 12. The tone of the referral was frustrated and angry, and the dietician cited "lack of cooperation and lack of progress." The dietician was answerable to a physician for her work with Sandra, which she felt was failing. In particular she blamed Sandra's mother, whom she stipulated as "overinvolved" with Sandra, and she felt family therapy was needed. The family arrived for the session and expressed confusion at the referral, but a willingness to be interviewed. The family consisted of mother, age, 30, father age 33, daughter, Sandra, age 12, and daughter, Ellen, age eight. The referral stated that Sandra was "anorectic," and that the family treatment was deemed necessary.

During the first interview, several salient issues emerged. To begin Sandra was far from "anorexic." Rather, she had unusual preferences that consisted of eating primarily french fries, bread and milk. She was small for her age, but had not experienced significant weight loss. Her ways of eating had been a problem to the family, and particularly to her mother, since she was an infant. Of importance for our purposes

GENOGRAM

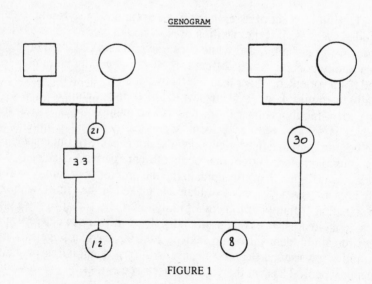

FIGURE 1

is that she had also been born with a severe congenital heart problem, surgically corrected one year ago. Her sister by comparison, was framed by the family as a very "good girl," who will "eat anything." Several issues and patterns emerged during the interview.

1. To begin, mother saw the problem as a huge problem. Father saw the problem as more minor. All agreed that mother was most worried, most upset, most concerned about the problem. The parents engaged in a complementary dance in which the more the father minimized the problem, the more the mother maximized the problem.
2. Mother and Sandra struggled daily over Sandra's eating. The struggles only occurred at dinner, the one meal when father was home. During other meals the girl was left alone to eat bread and milk. While mother and Sandra fought, father usually left the room and watched television.
3. The mother's mother believed the problem was a severe problem. She talked with her daughter frequently about it, and often sent her books and articles about anorexia. Conversely, the father's mother believed the problem was a minor problem, and told her daughter-in-law to leave Sandra alone. Thus, the struggle over definition of the problem and how to handle it, as seen in the parents was replicated in the two sides of the extended family. The interview revealed that a similar pattern had existed regarding Sandra's earlier heart problem, as mother and maternal grandmother showed worry, while father and paternal grandmother distanced.
4. Mother and her mother believed Sandra would stop eating altogether and would die in two or three years. Father's mother believed Sandra would begin to eat normally, on her own, in two or three years. In fact, Sandra was gradually eliminating foods that she would eat, thus adding to the mother's fear. Pushes from the dietician to increase her food intake and her food repertoire were met with Sandra eating less and less, replicating the family's complementary pattern.

Since the family had been referred by another professional, the dietician, it was decided to devote a portion of the interview to a family-larger system assessment, exploring the family's relationships with professional helpers. Several crucial factors emerged.

Due to Sandra's congenital heart problem the family had a long history with health professionals. Indeed, there was never a time in the life of the family when professional helpers were not engaged with it. A critical incident with the health care system emerged during this discussion.

> She was born with a congenital heart defect. I was seventeen at the time. The doctor came in and told me "Your baby has a heart problem" and then he said "Don't worry about it."

The mother's tone as she relayed this incident was one of frustration and near contempt. Her initial involvement with a health professional occurring as the family was forming left her feeling unsupported and misunderstood, mirroring her experience with both her husband and her father. She began to turn more and more to her mother for support. Both parents felt intimidated by Sandra's cardiologist. They lived for ten years waiting for Sandra to have open heart surgery, unsure of what questions to ask, and silently frightened that their daughter would not survive.

According to the mother, Sandra's eating problems developed in infancy and continued to the present. Frequently the mother would complain to her family physician (a second health professional) and ask for help. She commented that the eating problem was far easier to discuss and focus on than the heart defect. Also, she felt concerned that by eating poorly, Sandra's ability to survive surgery would be harmed, but when she raised this concern, it was dismissed by her husband and the doctor. According to mother, the physician's response was "leave her alone. She'll eat when she's hungry." Here, without realizing it, the physician had joined ranks with the husband and his mother, leading the wife to redouble her efforts to make Sandra eat. The effect of the outside helper's *inadvertent* alliance with father and grandmother contributed to the escalating and increasingly untenable struggle between mother and Sandra.

All direct involvements with outside helpers were the province of the mother (this is a very common situation, easily leading to the unintentional siding cited above.) The family supported this, as did the health care system by virtue of setting appointments when the father was unavailable, and never directly imparting information to him. Such involvement served to support the already problematic pattern of mother being more involved with the girl's eating, and father remaining aloof. Boundaries both in the family and between the family and helpers became skewed, such that information from both systems passed through mother, who was then eventually designated by the dietician as "overinvolved."

Following Sandra's successful recovery from serious heart surgery, the mother decided it was time to tackle her eating problem with professional help. Here, one may hypothesize that close involvement with outsiders from the health care system had become necessary and familiar to family functioning. Rather than reorganize without professionals, the family sought a new one in the dietician. Mother believed, however, that the referral to the dietician was simply the physician's way to "get her off his back." While remaining involved with health care professionals, the mother also expressed skepticism with their knowledge. Physicians had assured her of Sandra's future well-being after the heart surgery, but mother expressed a belief that Sandra would, in fact, cease eating altogether and die in a few years. She had never voiced this fear to the doctors, as she believed they would think she was foolish.

The dietician believed the problem was a very serious one. Her diagnosis of "anorexia" in a child who would eat half a loaf of bread for lunch, easily aligned her with the mother and her mother. Father discounted the dietician as a useful or necessary approach. Father's mother argued with her daughter-in-law regarding the necessity of professional help. *Now the professional network completely mirrored the family constellation*. Mother, her mother and the dietician believed Sandra had a serious, life-threatening condition, in need of immediate attention. Father, his mother, and the physician believed in backing off, and that Sandra would start to eat normally in time. Each position encouraged an exacerbation of the other position. Escalating complementarity pervaded the family-health care system. *The system was, in effect, paralyzed* (see Figure 2).

Exploration of the dietician's role with the family revealed that, like mother, she interacted primarily with Sandra. Mother and Sandra would go to the appointment together, but mother arranged for the dietician to see Sandra alone, out of the belief that Sandra would "open up" with her. Mother believed as many parents do, that the professional would be able to accomplish with she had not been able to do, namely, make Sandra eat. In point of fact, Sandra regarded the dietician with great derision, and the dietician, unknowingly, replicated mother's unsuccessful strategies. When asked about her visits to the dietician, Sandra replied with disgust, "she talks about Kiwi fruit."

Sandra emerged each week from the dietician's office with a list of two new foods to try. She handed this list to her mother, who then made a special trip to the store to purchase the items, thus involving her more in Sandra's unusual eating style. During this week, struggles

Family - Health Care System Triad

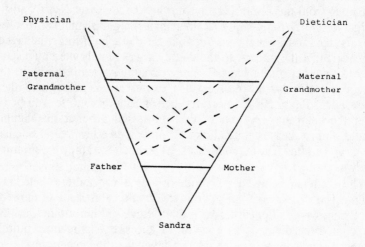

Key:
- - - - conflict
{   alliance
Complementary
Messages:

"Leave her alone -   "Make her eat"
she'll eat when she's ready"

"It's not a big problem"   "It's a big problem"

"No need for outside help"   "Go for help"

FIGURE 2

would then ensue, as mother attempted to get Sandra to eat the new items.

While the mother, by referral from the physician, had initiated the original contact with the dietician, and while she diligently shopped for items the dietician wanted Sandra to eat, she also found it impossible to carry out the dietician's instructions. At the point of referral to family therapy, the mother reported growing disenchantment with the dietician, and was following her instructions less and less. Nonetheless, she planned for Sandra to continue her weekly visits to the dietician.

The information generated in this interview about the family and multiple helpers aided me in a number of ways.

First, it was clear this was a system where the potential for triangulation of the therapist or *any* new health care provider, was rife. Father and mother, two grandmothers, and two professionals were aligned in perfect balance. A new ally for either side would temporarily tip the balance and likely result in the search for yet another helper by whichever side felt unsupported.

Second, since half the system appeared to believe that outside help was unnecessary, solutions that seemed to come from professionals ran the risk of discounting half the family.

Finally, the family had clearly tried various "common sense" solutions, such as the physician's advice to back off, and the dietician's advice to push Sandra to eat. None of these had worked, as they too closely mirrored the family's own struggle. The family, and mother, in particular, felt like failures, and anticipated criticism from professionals, as this had been implied in all earlier solution attempts.

This assessment of the family/mutual helpers system led me in several key directions that permeated the entire work with the family, and from which some lessons may be drawn, for work with other patients, their families, and the larger systems.

First, I maintained a stance of openness and curiosity in the relational domain, but refused to be drawn into the alliance patterns, I was careful neither to minimize the problem and thereby join father, nor maximize it and thereby join mother. This had the effect of beginning to put the parents on the same or symmetrical level, altering their previous complementary pattern.

The creation of an *unanticipated relationship* with a professional was further enhanced by the kinds of interventions utilized. All interventions were framed as "experiments" or "to gather information" rather than as proposed solutions. All interventions involved father, as well as mother. The father welcomed the opportunity to become involved, and began to speak about felling discounted in the past, but unable to enter because he felt "the doctors knew best." The parents were frequently encouraged to talk over and decide whether or not to do a particular "experiment," thus blocking credit to the therapist for any changes that might ensue, and, rather, placing ownership for changes within the family, while altering the family's prior complementary pattern *with helpers*, and replacing it with a symmetrical partnership.

Since the macrosystem had been permeated with advice-giving and implicit criticism, I chose to frame the parents as experts, citing their long experience with the health care system in their daughter's behalf. The parents began to really work together, and made a plan for Sandra. As they implemented the plan, becoming more assertive with Sandra and each other, they became more assertive with professionals. When the dietician countered their plan with one of her own, appointments with the dietician were stopped by both parents, and the family's boundaries vis-à-vis the health care system shifted profoundly. For the first time in the family's 12-year history with the health care system, they were invited to continually assess their child's progress. In short, a treatment partnership was formed, giving the family a very different relationship experience with a health care professional. The "news of a difference" at the macrosystemic level began to be replicated within the family, and the parents' formerly complementary relationship became more and more balanced and symmetrical. Sandra ceased being a "patient," began to eat normally and predictions of her death were replaced with predictions of her future life as a lawyer, drawing on what her father described as her special talent for "looking for loopholes!"

CONCLUSION

When a family system and the health care system first encounter one another, unacknowledged definitions of relationships are shaped, unspoken expectations are formulated, and unseen interactional patterns are set in motion.

The family system/health care system relationship is a co-created phenomenon, arising out of the historical contexts, beliefs, and daily operations of each system. Like other phenomena in effective patient care, however, its maintenance, its escalation into unfortunate patterns, and to generative recovery and healing can be powerfully effective by the steps taken by the health care system.

In "thinking systems," we are required to include ourselves, and not simply assess and intervene in the patient's family system.

Family-health care system interaction can be assessed briefly and can be utilized to orient the practitioner to work in innovative ways that avoid replicating both stuck family patterns and prior treatment failures.

Introducing aspects of symmetry into escalating complementary relationships or aspects of complementarity into ferocious symmetrical relationships between the family and health care system, avoiding un-

planned alliances and splits, realigning family-larger system boundaries, remembering that our theories are not the truth, (including this
one) and attending to widest possible context of multiple embedded
systems are our working tools, regardless of the specific content of
interventions. Presently, this complex relationship of family health
care systems is rarely addressed explicitly. Family-larger system interviews or work with families that address their relationship to the larger
systems as described above, are corrective efforts, taking place *after*
problems have ensued, and taken their toll on all concerned.

A preventive approach is crucial. Such prevention involves pre-ser-
vice and in-service training for health care providers that goes beyond
a discrete course in "family assessment" or "family interviewing."
Rather, an appreciation of complex systemic interaction is required
throughout a curriculum. Positive involvement and collaboration with
families at the initial onset of illness needs to occur through a combination of policy shifts in the health care system, the elaboration of new
norms and expectations, careful advocacy for families and their ill
members, and trained competency in macrosystemic process.

REFERENCES

Bloomfield, S., Nielson, S. & Kaplan, L. Retarded Adults, Their Families, and Larger Systems: A New role for the Family Therapist. In E. Imber-Coppersmith (Imber-Black) (Ed.),
Families With Handicapped Members. Rockville, Maryland: Aspen Systems Corporation,
1984, pp. 138-149.

Harlin, H.T. The Family and the Psychiatric Hospital. In J. Schwartzman (Ed.), *Families and
Other Systems: The Macrosystemic Context of Family Therapy*. New York: Guilford Press,
1985, pp. 108-132.

Imber-Coppersmith, E. (Imber-Black) The Family and Public Service Systems. In B. Keeney
(Ed.), *Diagnosis and Assessment in Family Therapy*. Rockville, Maryland: Aspen Systems
Corporation, 1983, pp. 83-99.

Imber-Coppersmith, E. Families and Multiple Helpers: A Systemic Perspective. In D. Campbell & R. Draper (Eds.) *Applications of Systemic Family Therapy*. London: Grune and
Stratton, 1985, pp. 203-212.

Sarason, S. & Doris, J. *Educational Handicap, Public Policy, and Social History: A Broad-
ened Perspective on Mental Retardation*. New York: The Free Press, 1979.

Schwartzman, J. Macrosystemic Approaches to Family Therapy. In J. Schwartzman (Ed.),
Families and Other Systems: The Macrosystemic Context of Family Therapy. New York:
Guilford Press, 1985, pp. 1-24.